I CAN MAKE YOU
THIN

LOVE FOOD,
LOSE WEIGHT

Also by Paul McKenna

CONTROL STRESS
I CAN MAKE YOU SLEEP
I CAN MAKE YOU RICH
QUIT SMOKING TODAY
INSTANT CONFIDENCE
CHANGE YOUR LIFE IN SEVEN DAYS
I CAN MEND YOUR BROKEN HEART (with Hugh Willbourn)
THE HYPNOTIC WORLD OF PAUL McKENNA

I CAN MAKE YOU
THIN

LOVE FOOD, LOSE WEIGHT

PAUL McKENNA Ph.D.

EDITED BY MICHAEL NEILL

BANTAM PRESS

LONDON · NEW YORK · TORONTO · SYDNEY · AUCKLAND

For Maureen Edwards

TRANSWORLD PUBLISHERS
61–63 Uxbridge Road, London W5 5SA
A Random House Group Company
www.rbooks.co.uk

I Can Make You Thin
first published in Great Britain
in 2005 by Bantam Press
an imprint of Transworld Publishers
Reissued 2007
90-Day Success Journal
first published in Great Britain
in 2006 by Bantam Press
This combined illustrated edition with new material
published in 2010 by Bantam Press

Art direction and design by Alex Tuppen. www.36studios.co.uk
Design and Artworking by Lynnette Eve. www.design-jam.co.uk

Illustrations on pages 118, 131 © Gillian Blease 2005, 2007, 2010
Photographs of Paul McKenna © Trevor Leighton
For other acknowledgements, see endmatter. Every effort has been made to obtain the necessary
permissions with reference to copyright material, both illustrative and quoted. We apologize for any omissions
in this respect and will be pleased to make the appropriate acknowledgements in any future edition.

A CIP catalogue record for this book
is available from the British Library.

ISBN 9780593064436

Addresses for Random House Group Ltd companies outside the UK
can be found at: www.randomhouse.co.uk
The Random House Group Ltd Reg. No. 954009

The Random House Group Limited supports The Forest Stewardship
Council (FSC), the leading international forest-certification organization. All our
titles that are printed on Greenpeace-approved FSC-certified paper carry the FSC logo.
Our paper procurement policy can be found at
www.rbooks.co.uk/environment

Printed and bound in Great Britain by Butler Tanner & Dennis Ltd, Frome

4 6 8 10 9 7 5

AN IMPORTANT NOTE FROM PAUL

How would you like to eat whatever you want whenever you want and still lose weight?

I know that seems like an outrageous claim, but it's true. Before long, you will be eating less and enjoying it more without feeling like you are missing out.

Since I wrote the original version of this book five years ago, I have learned even more about how to help people lose weight easily. My simple yet consistently effective approach has begun a revolution around the world, and what was once my lone voice in the wilderness has begun to become mainstream, as a growing army of scientists and doctors have been compiling more and more evidence that proves what I've known experientially for years:

Diets are the enemy of weight loss!

This system is so simple you will probably find it difficult at first to believe that it will work. That's because you have been brainwashed by diets into believing that weight loss is difficult, and it's not. In fact, two independent research studies into the effectiveness of my system have shown that what you are about to learn is seven times more successful than any diet!

Dieting has become a multi-billion-pound industry, and as a result of their approach, many of the people I talk to on my travels have been conditioned to feel stress every time they are around food, as if eating a piece of chocolate or a bowl of chips could cause them to balloon up to the size of a large blimp. I have actually seen people who won't walk into a room that has a buffet table because they feel so out of control in the presence of food.

My message is simple: Love food, lose weight!

That is why I have created this special edition of the book and filled it with images of so-called 'forbidden foods'. We are genetically programmed to enjoy eating, yet we've been taught that certain foods are bad for us and will make or keep us fat. It seems so unfair, and it would be – if it were true. This manufactured obsession with food is not only unhealthy, it's misleading. Food is not the enemy.

Every naturally thin person I have ever met eats a wide range of foods, including pizza, chips, ice cream and chocolate. Because their metabolisms have not been artificially slowed by years of dieting, they are able to eat what they want without losing control and without gaining weight. As you begin to use the 4 Golden Rules and listen to the mind-programming CD, your metabolism will reset to its natural speed and you will regain control.

Recently, a significant study into diets has been published which not only shows that they work for fewer than 10 per cent of the people who use them, but also that the vast majority of people who come off a diet end up putting on more weight than before they went on it. Diets are not just a symptom of the problem – they are significant part of its cause. I am completely serious when I say there is a better case for banning diets than banning smoking when we consider the health consequences to our nation.

Of course, nutrition matters when it comes to your body's health; but it has NOTHING to do with weight loss. In the past 50 years, there have been over 2,000 published diets and tens of thousands of recipes for 'weight loss' – and the world is fatter than it has ever been. The shifting sands of popular dieting fads tell you not to eat any carbs, or to eat less fat, or to eat different combinations of foods, and they all miss the point – when it comes to losing weight, **IT'S NOT ABOUT THE FOOD!**

It's the way you think and behave around food that makes the difference.

All your decisions about what you eat, when you eat and how much you eat take place in your mind. Using this system, together we are going to reprogram your mind to change the way you think about food forever. You will automatically start to feel more and more in control!

In this new and expanded edition of **I Can Make You Thin**, you will find the same ideas that have been used by over 5 million people to transform their relationship with food forever. I've added in a 90-day success journal and a quick-start DVD. If you're keen to get started, pop the DVD into your computer or DVD player and in less than half an hour you'll be on your way to a brand new you.

There are also a number of small but important changes, each one based on the fruits of my additional research and success with millions of people who've lost weight using my system. Especially important is the chapter that will show you how to overcome the single most difficult obstacle that stops people from making this system work for them – self-sabotage.

I've also added some more success stories and tips from people who've used the system successfully for themselves to impress upon you that once you know how, it really is easy to lose weight and keep it off for life.

Recently I met a lady who attended one of my seminars and lost a considerable amount of weight. She told me she was angry. When I asked her why, she said it was because she had spent years torturing herself with diets and feeling like a failure. In fact, she'd added up all the money she'd spent on diets, weight-loss programmes and special foods and it came to nearly ten thousand pounds. If only she'd known how easy weight loss really is, she could have saved herself all that money and years of unnecessary stress.

Much of what I am about to say will fly in the face of what you've done in the past and what you think is 'right'. You've tried other methods of weight loss and they didn't work or they only worked temporarily.

No matter what you've tried before, it's time to do something radically different . . .

To your good health,

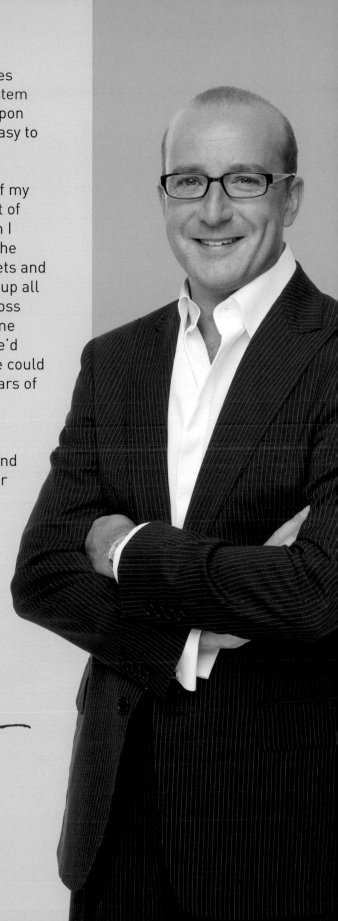

Paul McKenna

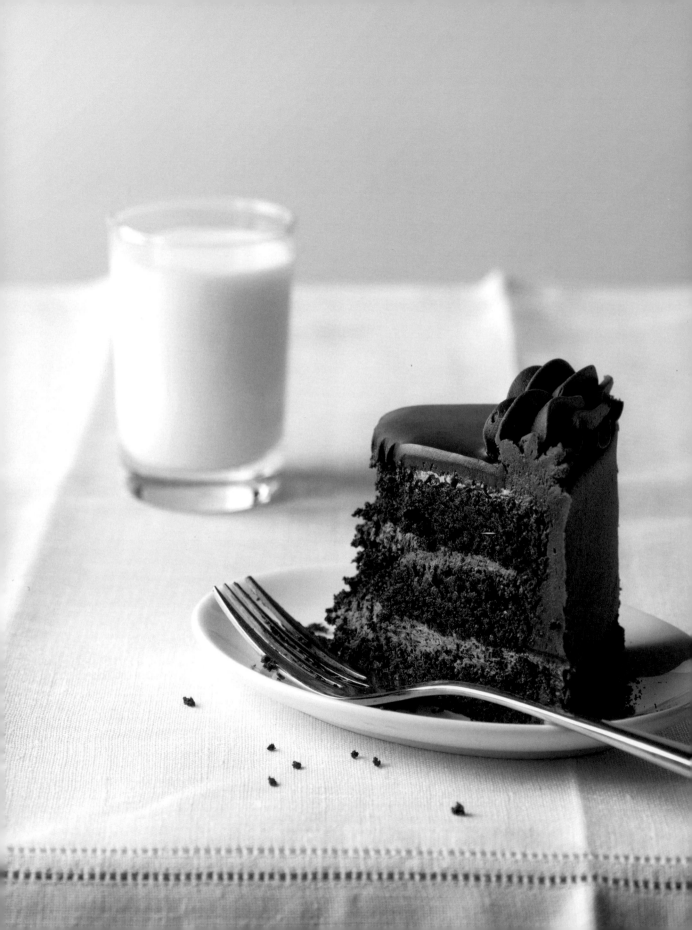

CONTENTS

PART ONE: I CAN MAKE YOU THIN

PART TWO: 90-DAY SUCCESS JOURNAL

PREFACE

As a medical nutritionist for more than two decades, I have seen patients lose weight on any number of diet programmes, then watched as they struggled to maintain their weight loss. The ability of overweight individuals to accept chronic food deprivation at levels as low as 400 calories a day for extended periods of time has never ceased to amaze me. Nor has the sad reality that most of them regain their hard-won losses. A significant number have undergone this process repeatedly.

Why couldn't obese individuals stay on a diet? Over the years, some patients told me that they just couldn't stop themselves. Others said they just ate mindlessly, often not knowing what they were eating. The common belief that eating is controllable has led us to expect people to 'behave' or pay the price of public shame. But diets don't work, eating is not due to lack of willpower. Eating, ultimately, is under the control of the brain.

In our world, where food is freely available, maintaining weight loss by dieting requires a continuous conscious effort to eat less. Like our inability to resist sleep, our brains will override our minds and make us eat. This is in the nature of any living organism where the brain dictates behaviour.

How can we alter this course? The answer lies not in the diet but in changing our response to signals from the brain. That is behaviour modification. In this book are all the keys to accomplishing that which seems impossible: losing weight and keeping it off.

No fad diets are recommended here; rather, an approach to controlling the response to hunger and, even more importantly, a way of altering the appetitive drive by reducing the stress that dieting causes.

This is a revolutionary approach and it is the only approach that will be successful long term without the use of medication. I recommend that the reader keep an open mind and closely follow the expert advice given here. This approach requires work, but in persistence will lie victory for those who have long fought this battle.

Ronald Ruden, M.D., Ph. D.
Lenox Hill Hospital, New York
Author of **The Craving Brain**

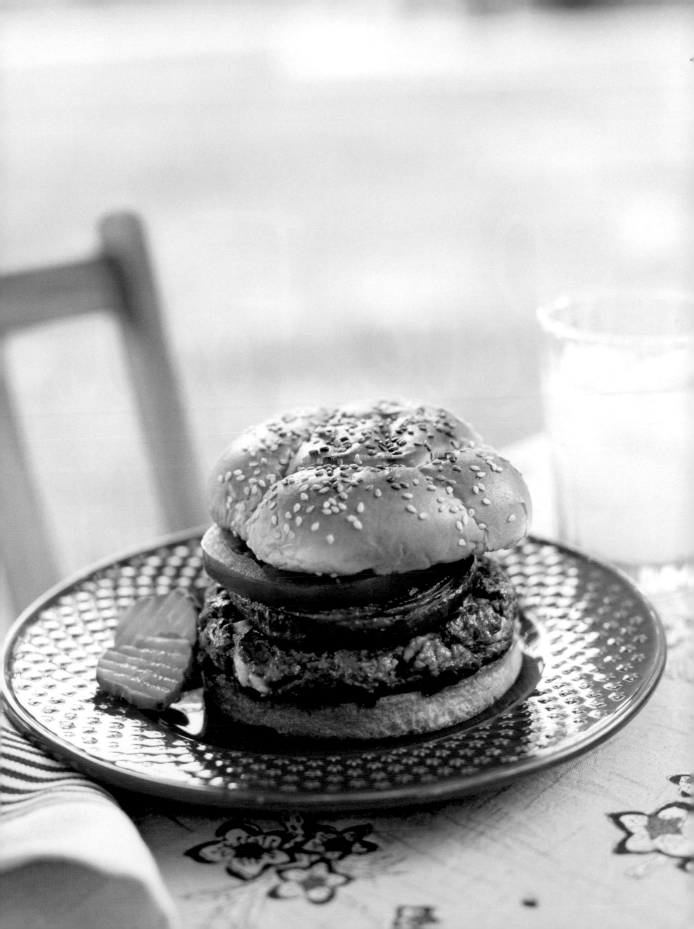

Love Food
Lose Weight

THE WEIGHT-LOSS MIND-PROGRAMMING CD

Your mind is like a computer – it has its own software, which helps you to organize your thinking and behaviour. Having worked with all sorts of people with different problems over many years, I have learned that almost all problems stem from the same cause: negative programs running in the unconscious mind.

This book comes with a powerful mind-programming CD that will fill your unconscious mind with positive willpower. While you become absorbed into a natural state of relaxation, I will reprogram your computer – your unconscious mind – so that you will change the way you think about food and feel better about yourself. I will give you suggestions that will help you to change your behaviour, eat better, speed up your metabolism and escape from the fixation with food.

It's best to listen to it when you have about half an hour where you can safely relax completely. As you listen to it regularly, you will reinforce all the changes you are making. In fact, it will make it much easier to stick to the golden rules I share with you in this book.

The latest research into the effectiveness of these and similar techniques has shown that listening to this CD over and over again, every day, will dramatically enhance your ability to lose weight. You don't have to believe it – just use it!

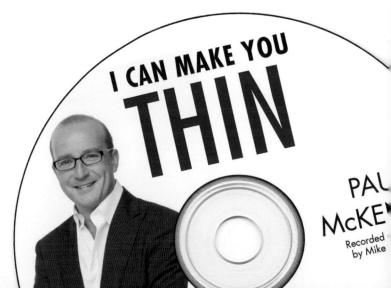

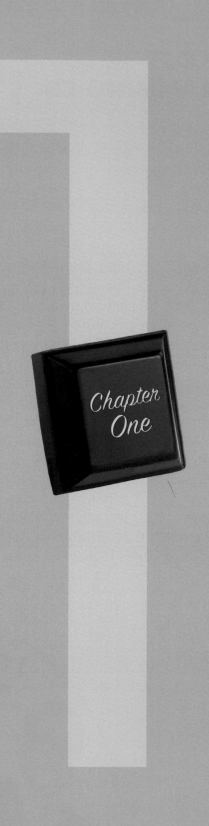

Chapter
One

ARE YOU READY FOR SOMETHING TRULY DIFFERENT?

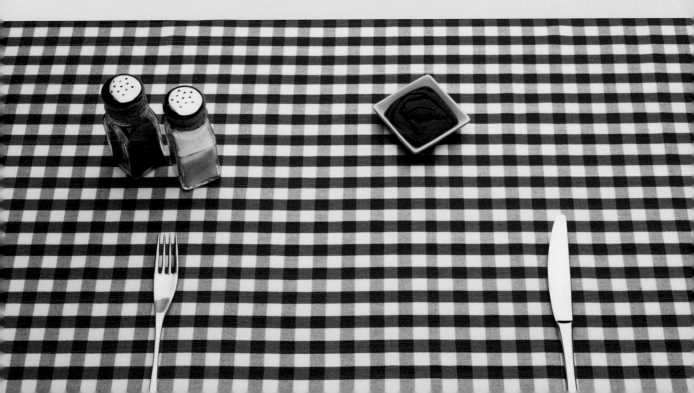

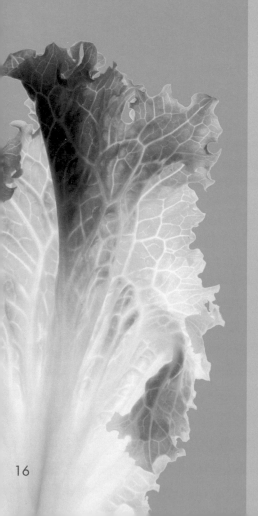

ARE YOU READY FOR SOMETHING TRULY DIFFERENT?

This may well be the easiest book on losing weight you have ever read. But don't be fooled by its simplicity. I have worked hard to make my system as concise as possible – so concise that you can probably understand the whole thing in less than a day. But what a day it will be!

During that time, you will not only discover what's been keeping you from the body you desire, but you'll also learn the simplest and most effective weight-loss system ever devised. It's a system that has helped people who felt as though they had failed at every diet in the world, or been overweight all their lives, as well as those people who just wanted to lose weight and feel great for life.

Whether your primary goal is to lose weight, lead a healthier lifestyle, feel really happy with your body or just to be able to shift those last ten pounds, then this system is exactly what you've been looking for!

I'll also reveal the truth about exercise and share with you some simple but powerful techniques to supercharge your metabolism, control your cravings and let go of the emotional issues you used to stuff down with food. Finally, I'll teach you some of my favourite mind-programming techniques, which you can use to feel better now and in the future; you'll be able to put on the CD any time you want to reinforce the principles deep into your unconscious mind.

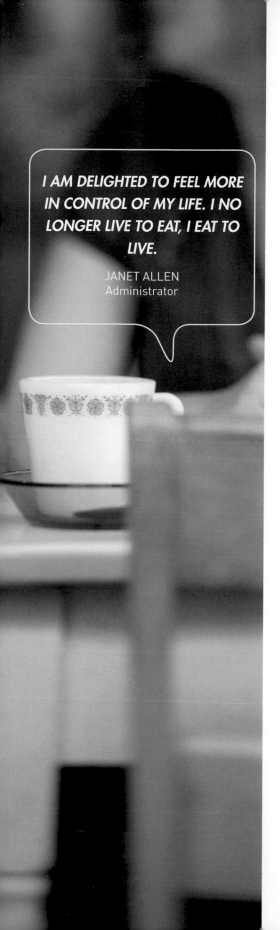

> *I AM DELIGHTED TO FEEL MORE IN CONTROL OF MY LIFE. I NO LONGER LIVE TO EAT, I EAT TO LIVE.*
>
> JANET ALLEN
> Administrator

But don't take my word for it – just follow my instructions step by step and notice how your body, and life, begin to change for the better.

LEARNING THE SECRETS OF NATURALLY THIN PEOPLE

Throughout the book, I will share with you the secrets that I have gleaned by studying naturally thin people. These are not the stick-figure models whose waif-like physiques come from eating disorders, drug addiction and airbrushing, but rather those people in life who somehow seem to be able to eat whatever they want and stay slim.

By developing the eating habits of naturally thin people, you'll be able to eat anything you want, whenever you want and still lose weight. Let's face it – you can have what you want, or you can have your reasons for not having it. So, if **absolutely anyone can lose weight with this system**, the only other question we need to ask is this:

Why aren't you thin yet?

There are three main patterns I have observed that keep people from living happily at their desired weight. As you read through the descriptions below, notice which of these apply to you. Then, when we begin reprogramming your mind in Chapter Three, you will be able to apply just the right tools and begin to lose weight immediately . . .

PATTERN ONE: OBSESSIVE DIETING

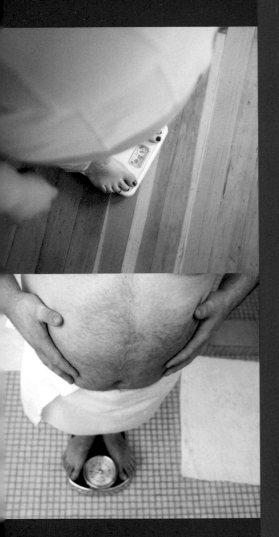

I was browsing through some of the recent releases in the weight-loss section of my local bookshop. What I found astounding was that despite the fact that nearly all of them were filled with 'forbidden food' lists, menus and calorie guides, they each began with the words 'This is NOT a diet'.

Let's begin by getting one thing straight:

A diet is any system of eating that attempts to exert external control over what, where, when or how much you eat.

Dieting has got a bad name over the past few years, and there's a good reason for that – scientific research shows that more than 90 per cent of people who attempt to lose weight by dieting fail.

Whenever somebody comes up to tell me about the weight they've lost on this great new diet, I ask them to come back and tell me about it in six months' time. If they are still happy about their weight and their diet in six months I am ready to listen. Unfortunately, I am still waiting for anybody to come back.

My theory? Too many diets, too few results. With over 25,000 diet books currently in print, many of which contain directly contradictory information, is it any wonder you find yourself as confused and misguided as the multi-billion-dollar weight-loss industry?

It's not just that diets don't work, many of them are an outright con. In fact, when I see celebrities who have 'battled their weight

FORGET ABOUT DIETING. FOR EVER. DIETS ARE ESSENTIALLY TRAINING COURSES IN HOW TO GET FAT AND FEEL LIKE A FAILURE.

problems' endorsing the latest fad diet, I don't know how they keep a straight face. In most instances, what they have actually done is tried a diet, lost weight and then put the weight back on again a few months later. Then they simply tried another diet, lost weight and promoted that one for a few months until the weight started piling back on.

In case you haven't picked up on the message here, it's this:

Forget about dieting. For ever. Diets are essentially training courses in how to get fat and feel like a failure.

The more diets people try and fail at, the more they convince themselves that they will never be able to lose weight. What nobody tells you is that the real reason most weight-loss programmes don't work is nothing to do with you – it's to do with human biology.

In his seminal study into human starvation during the Second World War, biological researcher Ancel Keyes discovered that reducing people's diet to a state of semi-starvation produced symptoms of irritability, loss of endurance and obsessive behaviour around food, including but not limited to lying, hoarding and stealing.

Even more telling, in the three-month period after the semi-starvation was ended and people could once again eat whatever they wanted, their obsession with food continued. Many people ate up to eight times as much food as they had done before the study began. (Does any of this sound familiar?)

That experiment, documented in the 1950s treatise **The Biology of Human Starvation,** is considered unreplicable. After all, to purposely starve people would be cruel and inhumane. But here's an interesting fact: the semi-starvation rations from the original study amounted to about 1,500 calories a day – more than is allowed in any number of the thousands of diets currently in vogue.

What all this goes to show is that depriving yourself of food is the worst possible way to lose weight. And if what you're doing isn't working, you need to do something different.

PATTERN TWO: EMOTIONAL EATING

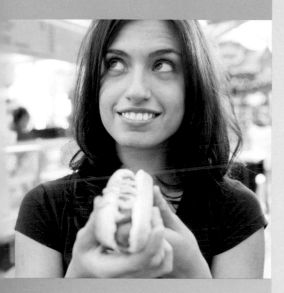

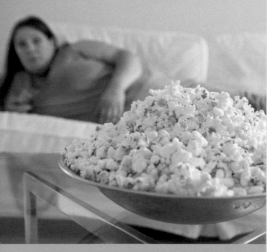

I am convinced that after diets, emotional eating is the number-one cause of obesity in the world. Many times people eat because they are bored or lonely or miserable or tired, or any one of a hundred emotional reasons, none of which has anything to do with physical hunger. If you eat based on emotional hunger, your body will never feel satisfied by food. This is why many people think that they never feel full – they never get the signal to stop eating because they were never hungry for food in the first place.

Maybe you first put on weight following a trauma or difficult time in your life and you began to comfort eat to help you through that time. Now, even though that stressful time is past, you have kept the dysfunctional habit of eating when you feel upset, lonely or just bored. This habit stems from a fundamental misunderstanding of why we feel what we feel.

An emotion is a bit like someone knocking on your door to deliver a message. If the message is urgent it knocks loudly; if it's very urgent it knocks very loudly; if it is very urgent and you don't answer the door, it knocks louder and louder and louder until you open the door or it breaks it down. Either way, the emotion will continue to come up until it's done its job. As soon as you 'open the door' by listening to the emotional message and taking appropriate action, the emotion will simply go away.

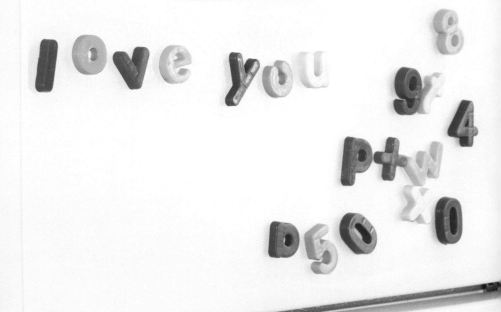

The good news is that with this new understanding, you don't have to be a victim any more. While I will be sharing a number of powerful techniques in the chapter on Emotional Eating, one of my colleagues has achieved an extraordinary amount of success simply by making his clients put a giant question mark on their fridge. The question mark is there to remind them to stop before grabbing a snack and ask themselves this question:

Am I really hungry, or do I just want to change the way I feel?

If it turns out that what you actually want is a change in the way you feel, no amount of food will work as well as applying the simple techniques in this book and on the mind-programming CD.

ONE ADDITIONAL THOUGHT

I am continually surprised at the number of women (and occasionally men) I work with who realize that their initial weight gain coincided with a traumatic incident from the past, ranging from episodes of sexual abuse to seemingly innocuous teasing leading to embarrassment in front of their peers.

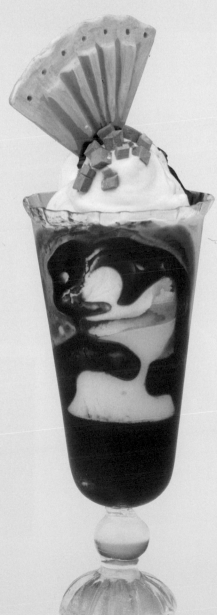

While the techniques in this book and on the mind-programming CD will help, they are not intended as a substitute for professional guidance. If you suspect this could apply to you, speak to your doctor and ask them to recommend an appropriate therapist.

PATTERN THREE: FAULTY PROGRAMMING

If you are overweight it's not your fault – it's the natural result of your current mental programming, and no diet, pill, shake or 'how-to' book can change that. The only way to lose weight and keep it off is to go to the unconscious mind and change your relationship with food for ever.

So relax. You are not crazy, you are not broken and you are not a bad person. You have simply developed some very unproductive habits. The good news is that once you learn to reprogram your mind, it will be just as simple to develop new habits of thinking and acting that will guarantee your success.

You don't even have to believe that it will work. Just follow my instructions and you will not only lose weight but stop obsessing about food for ever.

In just a few minutes, I'm going to share with you the four most important things you will ever learn about losing weight and keeping it off for life. But before we get started I want you to stop for a moment and do the following thought experiment . . :

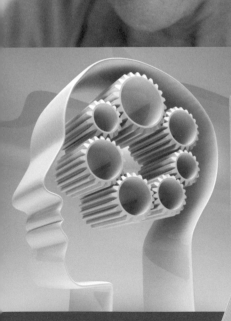

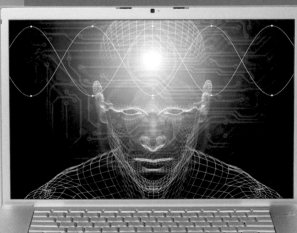

THE POWER OF PERSPECTIVE

Go to near the end of your life. Imagine that it is many years from now and you decided NOT to follow my instructions and begin losing weight. Instead, you carried on trying one diet after another, continuing to gain weight and lose your precious vitality year after year after year . . .

- **What were the consequences of that decision on your health?**

- **What were the consequences on your relationships?**

- **What were the consequences on your sense of wellbeing?**

- **How do you feel in your body?**

Now . . . take a few moments to imagine following this program and easily reaching and maintaining your target weight.

- **How good does this feel?**

- **How much energy do you have?**

- **What are you able to do?**

- **What clothes are you able to wear?**

- **Who are you with? What are you doing? (Besides that . . .)**

- **Exactly what will it be like when you have lived at your target weight for years and years?**

Now . . . STOP!

It's time to decide. If you want to hang on to your excuses and your excess weight, you may as well put the book down now.

But if you're ready finally to get that monkey off your back (and those inches off your waist), know that what you do from this moment onwards is entirely up to you. So let's get started!

MICHELLE HINES

The fat girl is five years and 140 pounds ago. I didn't love her nearly as much as I love the new, improved, thin me. Being fat isn't being happy.

My life was one food obsession after the other: cabbage soup, points, calories, fat, fibre, vinegar, whatever magic potion I could find; always on the quest for that elusive miracle that would cause me to one day wake up thin. Something that I didn't have to pay attention to, something that would change my life.

I was a chubby kid, a fat teen and fatter adult. The battle with weight began when I was very young, around nine years old; my mother thought I was too big and a consultation with the family doctor had me on a restrictive diet and prescription drugs. The only lesson I learned was to conceal the food I was eating. And the food was always in control; I never knew how to say no to it. I never felt satisfied. No matter how much I wanted to radiate health in a body that made me proud, I didn't know how. Until I found my miracle: Paul McKenna.

I don't know what happy twist of fate led me to the book/CD that at the time was only available in the UK, but I'm

forever grateful. Thanks to **I Can Make You Thin**, being healthy and at a good weight have become second nature, like breathing. I've never in my life felt this free. The ability to recognize when I'm full and stop eating is a precious and liberating gift. To know that I can eat French fries if I want them, enjoy them fully when I do indulge, but also to choose a healthy lifestyle, is profound and sublime. I have never, ever before in my life felt this wellness, this vitality.

Often when people talk to me about my lifestyle changes, they'll say, 'I know it's hard' or, 'It's always a battle.' And now I say, no, it's not. It's easier than anything I've ever done before. I didn't just change my weight, I changed my relationship with food. My life, my perspective, my moods, my body: everything improved.

I look at my before photo and wonder who that girl was. She seems so distant to me, and yet she's an important part of my past. I just wonder why I let her stay so unhappy for so long. But she helps me appreciate the woman I am now. Shopping for clothes is a joy, and far fewer photos of me end up in the trash bin. I have fallen in love with a new way of living.

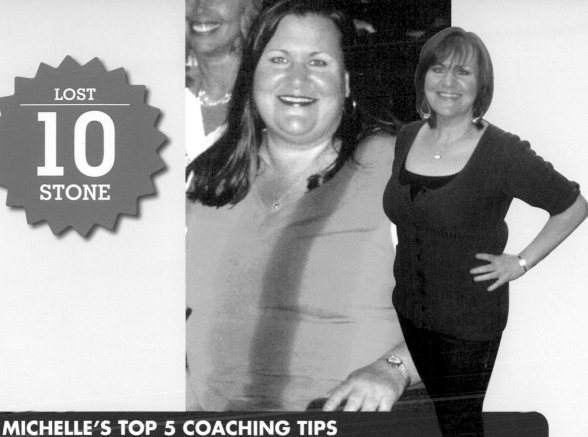

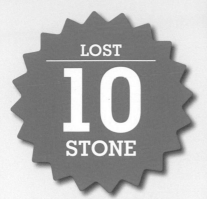

LOST
10
STONE

MICHELLE'S TOP 5 COACHING TIPS

1 **Listen to the CD every day.** I made the commitment to listen at least five days a week, and I kept to it for a year. After that, most of the weight was gone!

2 **Get rid of your fat clothes as you start wearing smaller sizes.** This was very challenging for me at first, but in my heart and soul I knew that I'd changed.

3 **Be prepared for profound changes in the way you feel about yourself.** I didn't know how unhappy I was until I said goodbye to all that fat.

4 **One of Paul's most useful tools is to put your utensils down between every bite of food.** This is second nature to me now.

5 **Educate yourself a little about the food you eat.** I love the way I feel when I eat healthy foods. That's a profound gift: it's easy to choose good food! I always wanted to know what it was like to be the girl who'd keep a pack of M&Ms on her desk and make it last for days – now I know, but I truly don't care for M&Ms any more!

FREQUENTLY ASKED QUESTIONS ABOUT 'ARE YOU READY FOR SOMETHING TRULY DIFFERENT?'

 I've tried lots of different ways to lose weight and none of them have worked. How is your system different?

In a fascinating study at the University of Hertfordshire, Professor Ben Fletcher achieved spectacular results by teaching people to respond to their 'hunger pangs' by going out and doing something in the world – turning off the TV and going for a walk, speaking to a friend or even going out to a movie. As a result of 'doing something different' around food, their habits began to change. People naturally began to make healthier choices about food and exercise.

The reason nothing's worked before is you've done the same thing over and over again – you've systematically starved yourself by dieting. The only thing you've changed is the recipes. And the definition of insanity is doing the same thing and expecting a different result!

 What if I'm really overweight – can I still use this system or do I need to diet first?

This system is directly at odds with any and every diet you might try, because it is diets and the dieting mentality that were making and keeping you overweight in the first place!

At the risk of repeating myself, I'll say it one more time:

Anything or anyone who tries to tell you what, where, when or how much to eat is teaching you to ignore your body – and if you're overweight, your body is trying to tell you it doesn't like being ignored!

I don't care how much you weigh, if you've been overweight all your life or if all your family are overweight – as you use this system you will lose weight and feel more in control and better about yourself.

Q. How well does this work? I want to look like the models in magazines . . .

So do the models in the magazines. Most of the pictures you see on magazine covers have been digitally altered in order to make the cover striking so that you will buy the magazine. They are not representative of reality.

Rather than compare yourself to something that doesn't exist, it's far better to compare yourself to yourself. Far too many women compare themselves with an airbrushed picture of an anorexic girl on a magazine cover and decide they aren't good enough as a human being. You are likely to feel significantly better if you ask yourself this question instead:

How much better am I getting?

Actually, I lived in New York for a number of years and had the opportunity to meet many of the world's most famous models. What struck me was that even though many of these women looked incredibly beautiful, they were pretty miserable, which I suppose is understandable given that they're so hungry all the time! I realized that they spent all their time looking for flaws and rarely saw the perfection of who they already were.

As the great poet Goethe said, 'It's not so important where we stand but the direction in which we are moving.' Human beings are usually at any time either getting better or worse. If you are getting better, excellent. If you are getting worse, then you know the direction in which you need to move.

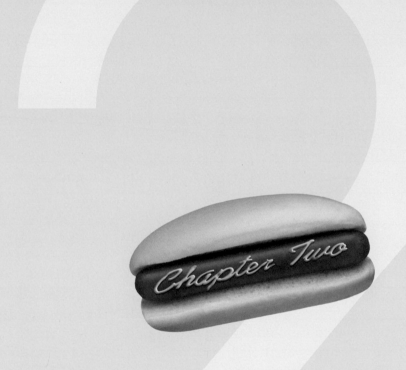

Chapter Two

THE SIMPLEST WEIGHT LOSS SYSTEM IN THE WORLD™

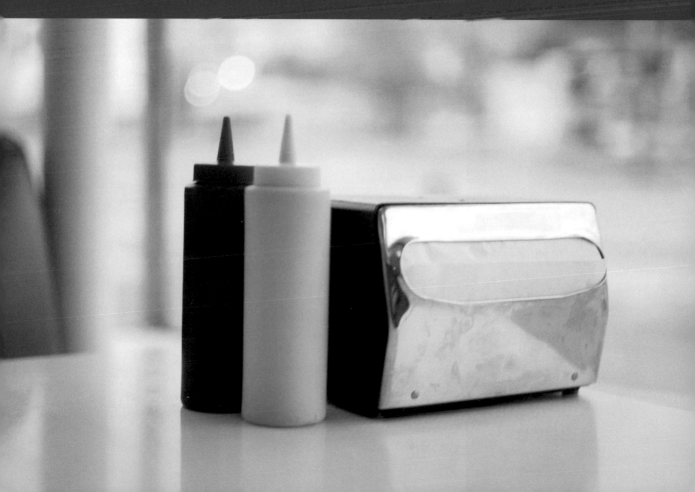

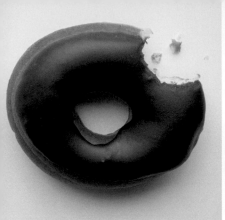
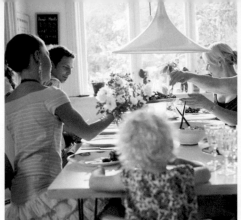
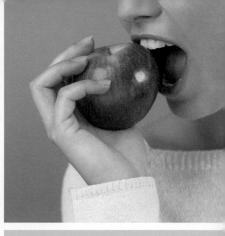
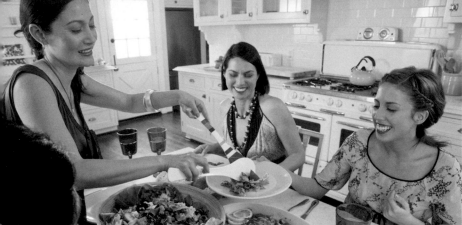

I GOT FED UP WAKING EVERY MORNING OBSESSING ABOUT FOOD. SINCE I STARTED USING PAUL'S SYSTEM, I DON'T. IT'S GREAT!

JANET COBB, TRAINER

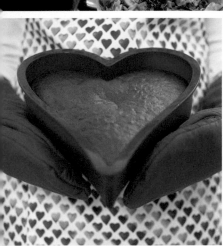
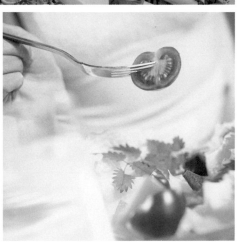
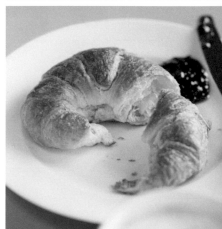
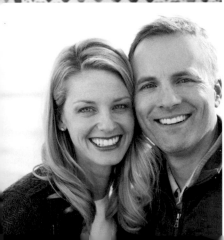
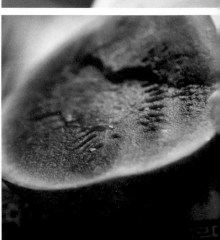

THE 'SECRETS' OF NATURALLY THIN PEOPLE

4 GOLDEN RULES

1 **WHEN TO EAT**

2 **WHAT TO EAT**

3 **HOW TO EAT IT**

4 **HOW MUCH TO EAT**

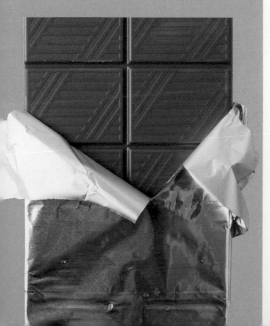

Sometimes people ask me how I came up with this system. Was I ever overweight myself? Did I study physiology at university? Did I just conjure it up out of thin air?

The reality is, it's taken me over fifteen years to develop this system and refine it to the point where I can share it with you today in the pages of a book. Over that time, I compared the mindsets and strategies of chronically overweight people with those who seemed to be 'naturally thin'.

What I discovered is that there are no 'naturally thin' people – it's just that some people were fortunate enough not to have been brainwashed by diets and the weight-loss industry into ignoring their bodies and blindly following the medical establishment, many of whom are funded by the very weight-loss industry they so heartily recommend.

Your body is smarter than any diet on earth, but with volumes of information all around us about how the 'wrong' foods will adversely affect our health or make us put on weight, it can be difficult to see, hear or feel what your body is telling you. That's why what I am about to explain to you is all you really need to change the way you eat for ever.

The real secret of being naturally thin is simply to introduce four new habits into your life – four 'golden rules' for deciding when to eat, what to eat, how to eat it and how much of it to have. These small habits will make a huge difference in your life – four simple guiding principles that will help you to make the best food choices in any situation you may encounter . . .

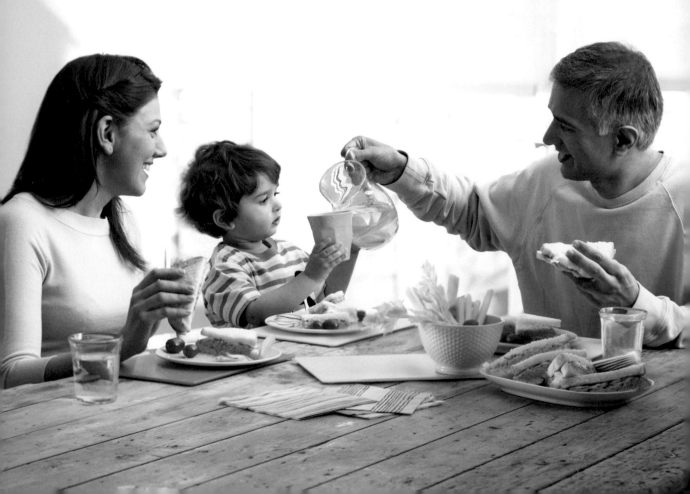

GOLDEN RULE NUMBER **1**

WHEN YOU ARE HUNGRY,

EAT

HOW STARVING YOURSELF CAN ACTUALLY MAKE YOU FAT

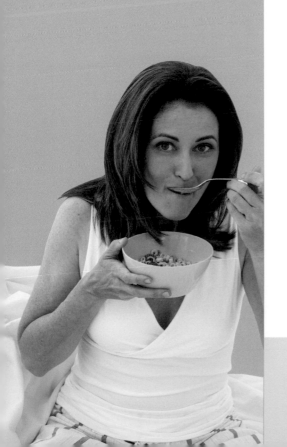

PAUL MCKENNA'S WEIGHT-LOSS SYSTEM IS THE BEST THING I HAVE EVER DONE.

PETER WILKINSON, DESIGNER

Ever wondered what's inside a camel's hump? It's fat – stored fat. Camels store fat because they don't know how long they're going to go between meals. When you starve yourself by not eating when you're hungry, your body does the same thing. In fact, if you've been trying to lose weight for a while, your body is probably stuck in continual fat-storage mode. It thinks there is a famine, and in response it goes into survival mode and stores fat in your cells, 'just in case'. Over time, your body begins to leach more fat from whatever foods you do eat. There may be only a few grams of fat in that 'Weight Watchers' lasagne, but if you're eating at 'mealtimes' instead of when you're hungry, your body will do whatever it takes to grab that fat and put it where it can store it until later – generally your stomach if you're a man and your hips and thighs if you're a woman.

That's partly why thin people can eat a lot and not put on weight – they aren't starving themselves so their bodies can either make use of or easily eliminate excess fat from their food.

In addition, consistently overriding your body's natural call for food alters your metabolism. A faster metabolism burns more calories throughout the day, but when you stop yourself from eating when you're hungry, your metabolism slows down so your body can conserve energy. This leads to feelings of lethargy, which many people experience as a mild depression.

If all that wasn't enough, not eating when you're hungry sets up dysfunctional patterns of thinking in the unconscious mind in relation to food. This subtle tension around food sets up a powerful neurochemical change in the brain that leads to false hunger signals and patterns of craving and bingeing. The vicious cycle is in motion – the less you trust your body, the less trustworthy your body's messages become.

There is, however, some very good news:

All you need to do to reset your body's innate wisdom is to eat whenever you feel truly hungry.

True hunger is different from emotional hunger (which we will deal with in Chapter Four). If you read the first golden rule and said to yourself, 'But I'm hungry all the time!' or even 'But I'm never hungry!', chances are what you're experiencing is more emotional than physical. Fortunately, as soon as you begin to listen to your body, you will once be able to easily recognise the subtle and not so subtle signs of true, authentic hunger.

At this point I want to introduce you to an amazing tool that you can use to know exactly when to start eating and when to stop. I call it the hunger scale.

The hunger scale goes from one, which is physically faint with hunger, to ten, which is stuffed to the point of nausea.

Take a few moments right now to look at the hunger scale and tune in to your body. How hungry are you right now?

Each person is different, but as a general rule, you'll want to eat whenever you notice yourself between 3 and 4 on the scale – that is, when you are fairly hungry, but before you become ravenous. If you wait until you get down to 1 or 2, your body will go into starvation mode and you'll wind up probably eating more than your body needs and storing the excess as fat.

Of course, if you have been a serial dieter you may be so used to overriding your body's signals that you might at times 'forget to eat' until you're already ravenous. If you think this might be you, practise tuning in to your body once an hour and giving yourself a number from 1 to 10 until you begin to notice differences between different points on the scale.

The more you practise tuning in to your own hunger, the sooner you'll be able to recognize your body's subtle signals long before your stomach growls and your brain starts to get fuzzy.

THE HUNGER SCALE

HOW HUNGRY ARE YOU RIGHT NOW?

1. **Physically faint**
2. **Ravenous**
3. **Fairly hungry**
4. **Slightly hungry**
5. **Neutral**
6. **Pleasantly satisfied**
7. **Full**
8. **Stuffed**
9. **Bloated**
10. **Nauseous**

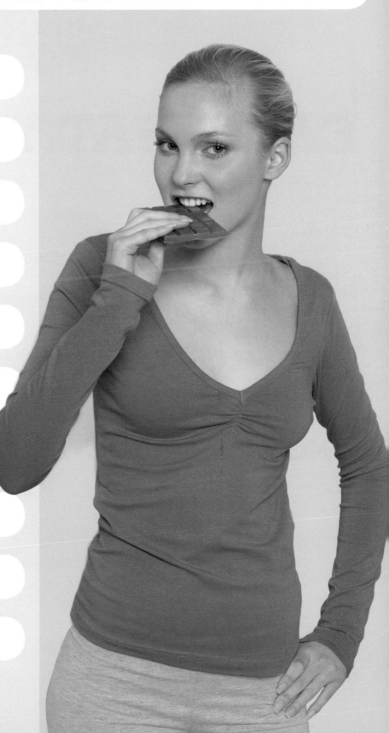

GOLDEN RULE NUMBER 2

EAT WHAT YOU WANT,

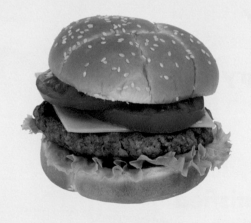

NOT WHAT YOU THINK YOU SHOULD

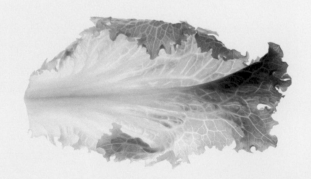

RESISTANCE IS FUTILE

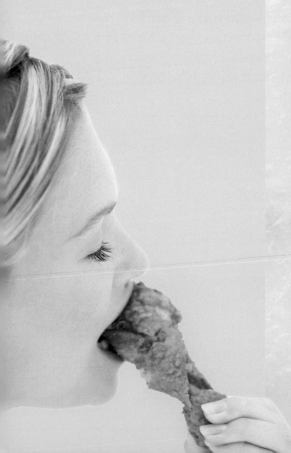

In a fascinating experiment performed in the 1930s, scientists gave a group of toddlers unlimited twenty-four/seven access to a vast range of foods from ice cream to spinach, essentially allowing them over a period of thirty days to create their own diet based on their own sense of what they wanted to eat and when.

The result?

While they each chose different foods at different times, every single child in the study wound up eating what was considered to be a balanced diet over the course of the month.

Similarly, many women have had the experience of unusual food cravings during pregnancy. The reason a pregnant woman will crave everything from ice cream to pickled onions is that her body is telling her exactly what it needs from moment to moment to 'build a baby'.

But as soon as you tell yourself not to eat certain foods (usually because you've been told they're bad for you), you upset the natural balance of your relationship with them. Rather than wanting it less, that 'forbidden food' instantly becomes more attractive to you. The inner battle between your positive intention and your resistance to being controlled (even by yourself) can be exhausting. As you begin to make peace with food and learn to listen to the wisdom of your body, you experience freedom from the tension and guilt that come from NOT following your intuition.

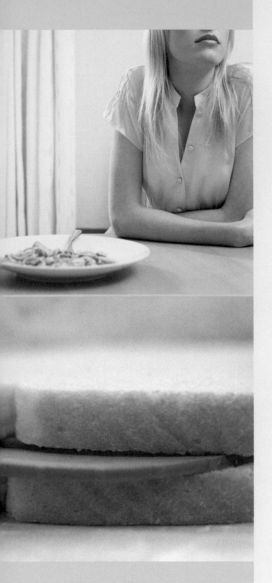

This is why there are NO forbidden foods in my system – you can eat anything you want any time you are hungry, providing you take the time to really, really enjoy it (see Golden Rule Number 3!).

In fact, why not go one step further?

You may in the past have been on one diet or another that told you to empty your cupboards of any foods high in fat, sugar, carbohydrates or whatever food you were being forbidden to eat.

My instructions for you are radically different.

Today, as soon as you finish reading this book, I want you to go to your refrigerator and throw out any food that does not totally inspire you to eat it. Chuck the diet soda. Throw out the low-fat yogurts. Unless you absolutely love them, bin the sugar-free popsicles. You'll know that you're done when there isn't a single thing in your fridge that you wouldn't be delighted to eat – and when you're next hungry, that's exactly what I'm asking you to do.

Fancy a bit of pasta?

Go for it.

Cake and ice cream calling to you?

As long as you're actually hungry, enjoy, enjoy, enjoy.

From this day forward, nothing is off-limits to you. Ever.

And if you really want to say 'NO' to something, say it to the purveyors of sugar-free low-carb cardboard-tasting crap.

NO FORBIDDEN FOODS

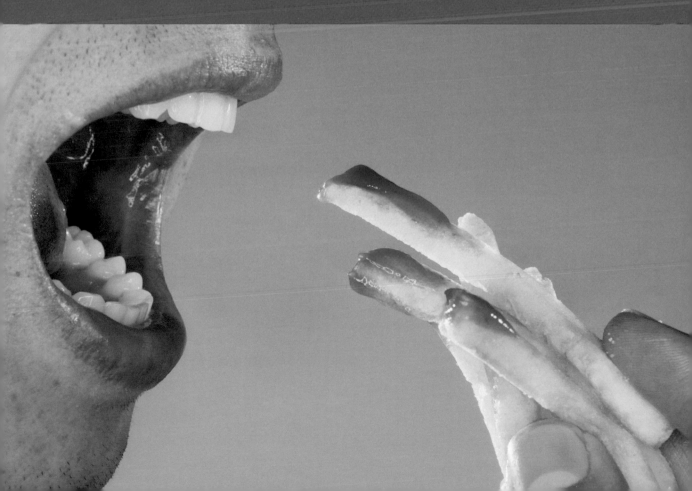

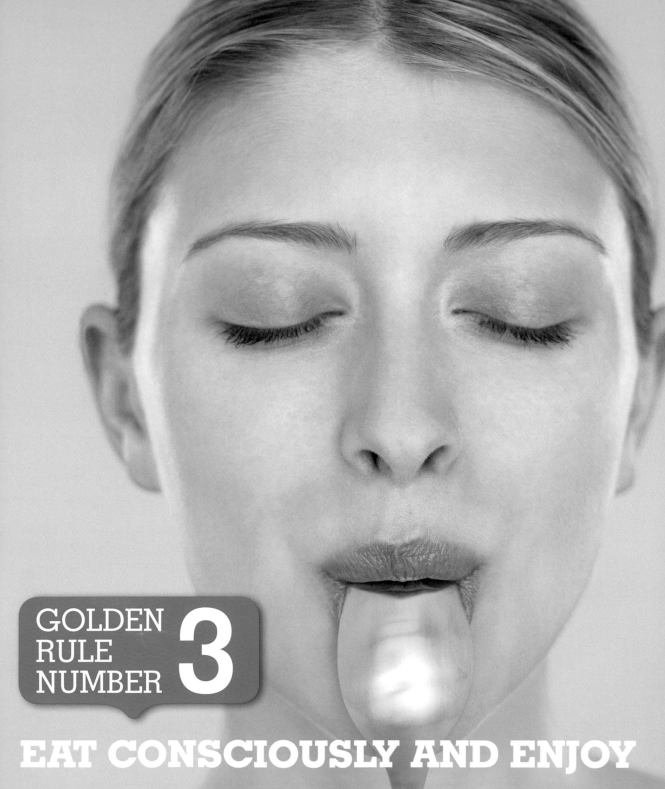

GOLDEN RULE NUMBER **3**

EAT CONSCIOUSLY AND ENJOY
EVERY MOUTHFUL

CONSCIOUS EATING

> ## PAUL'S SYSTEM HAS CHANGED ME. I HAVEN'T EATEN CHOCOLATE SINCE I STARTED USING IT.
>
> ELAINE HOPKINS, ADMINISTRATOR

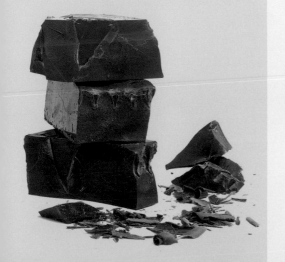

I've noticed a funny thing about people who are overweight. They spend all their time thinking about food – except when they're actually eating it. Then they go into a kind of 'eating trance', where they shovel as much food into their mouths as fast as they can without actually chewing or tasting anything.

Strange as it may seem, there is a very good reason for that. Whenever we do something that is essential for our survival, like eating, breathing deeply or making love, we release a 'happy chemical' in our brains called serotonin.

People who are overweight often shovel food into their mouths as quickly as possible in order to get a serotonin high. Unfortunately, because they are eating unconsciously, they never notice the signal from their stomach that lets them know they are full. So they keep on stuffing their faces, expanding their stomachs and putting on weight.

The problem is that even though they feel temporarily high from cramming in lots of food, they feel fat and guilty afterwards. In fact, they feel so bad that they repeat the whole ritual of unconsciously stuffing themselves again in order to anaesthetize the bad feelings they just created!

One of the unique features on my weight-loss programme is this:

You can eat whatever you want, whenever you want, so long as you fully enjoy every single mouthful.

I cannot emphasize this enough. I mean really enjoy it – savour the taste and enjoy the wonderful textures and sensations as you thoroughly chew each mouthful. Of course, in order to fully enjoy your food you have to notice that you're eating it.

I remember seeing a friend of mine who had lost a ton of weight and looked amazing. When I asked her how she had done it, she told me she had just returned from a luxury health resort in the Far East that cost £1,000 a day. When I asked what was the basis of the weight-loss regime they had used, she explained that, in the West, we eat far too fast.

At the spa, they taught her to slow her eating speed and become more conscious of the process of smelling, tasting and chewing her food. Each meal was like a meditation, and to help her to remember to do it, the spa assigned someone to sit opposite her during every meal and constantly remind her to slow down and savour each mouthful.

To put it to work for you, here is one simple thing you can do to help create enjoying each mouthful as a new and positive habit:

For the next two weeks, slow your eating speed down to about a quarter of what it used to be and chew each mouthful thoroughly.

It's very important to put your knife and fork down between every mouthful, so you can give your body time to notice what it's doing. Of course, if you're not using cutlery, prise your fingers off your sandwich and put it down between each mouthful. When your mouth is empty, you can pick up where you left off.

In this way, you make every bite a conscious choice, eating your food like a gourmet and savouring every mouthful instead of shovelling it in on automatic like a barnyard animal.

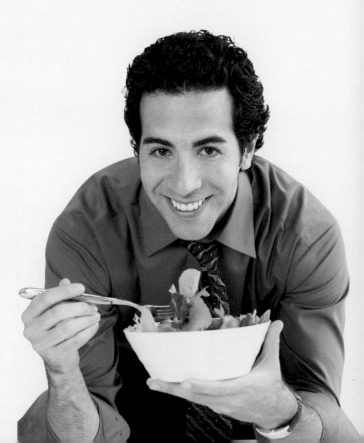

THE IMPORTANCE OF ELIMINATING DISTRACTIONS

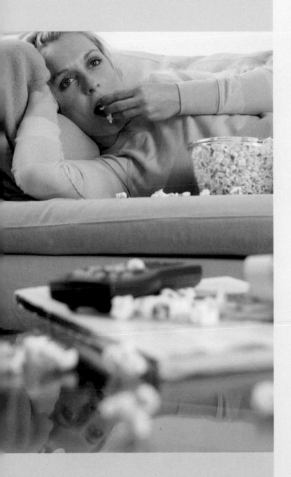

Of course, eating consciously does not only mean eating slowly. Until you really get the hang of this system, it means concentrating on your food and nothing else. A recent study conducted in Switzerland showed that when people were blindfolded, they ate 25 per cent less than when they could see – in other words, when they weren't looking at the food but were instead totally concentrating on the taste and texture, they actually ate less.

This corresponds with what I've noticed on my weight-loss seminars. After lunch, people will often report that their food tasted amazing, because for the first time in ages they were eating slowly and consciously enough to actually taste it and notice the feeling of being full.

Professor Brian Wansink, author of the amazing book **Mindless Eating**, has conducted some extraordinary experiments that show conclusively that when we are distracted during the process of eating, we not only don't notice what we are eating, we eat substantially more of it.

You can probably remember for yourself a time when you were eating popcorn, nuts or crisps while watching a film or a football match. By the time you 'woke up' and came to your senses, the entire bowl, bag or packet was gone, no matter how hungry you were when you started.

Since studies show that a whopping 91 per cent of people eat in front of the television, a powerful way to begin disrupting your old unconscious habits is to simply stop eating while reading, chatting on the phone or watching the telly. By eliminating as many distractions as possible while you eat, at least when you are first learning this system, you will find it considerably easier to notice and apply the fourth golden rule . . .

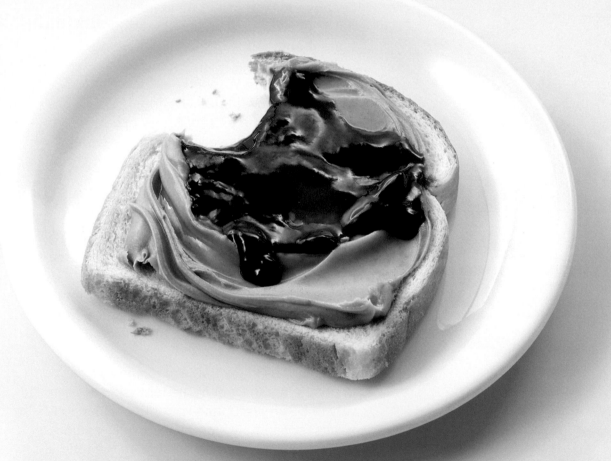

YOUR INNER THERMOSTAT

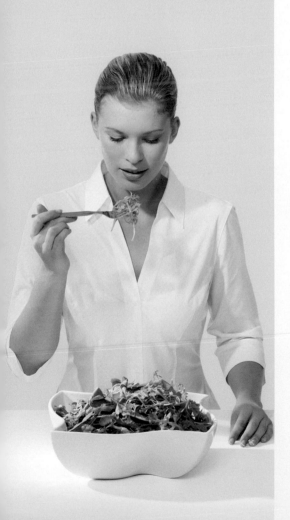

I remember as a kid using my mother's kettle to steam open an envelope. In order to keep the steam rising, I had to hold the 'on' switch down long after the kettle had boiled. Of course, kettles aren't designed to be used that way, and soon the metal thermostat inside the kettle became bent and stopped working properly.

Fortunately, it was quite easy to fix. All I had to do was go inside and bend the thermostat back into place. Immediately, the kettle began working perfectly again.

The natural design of the human body is to eat when we're hungry and stop when we're satisfied, but many of us are conditioned to eat until we think we're full – or even worse, until whatever food we put on our plate is gone.

To lose weight effortlessly and keep it off, you must begin working with your body and not against it. To get slim and stay slim we need to re-sensitize ourselves to our 'inner thermostat' so we can stop eating when we are full and feel good for the rest of the day.

In reality, when you've eaten enough, your stomach sends a signal – a sensation that says, 'I'm satisfied – that's enough.'

Although studies have shown that it can take up to twenty minutes for that signal to reach your brain, when you slow down your eating speed and eat more consciously, it becomes easier and easier to notice this signal as soon as it's sent. Most people experience it as a gentle, clear, satisfied sensation in their solar plexus (the area below your ribcage but above your stomach).

Even if you miss this warm feeling of satisfaction when it first occurs, there's another way to know that your stomach is full. As soon as you've had enough to eat, you'll notice that each subsequent bite of food becomes a little less enjoyable than the one before. The more you pay attention to this phenomenon, the more obvious it becomes.

Since continuing to eat after this satisfied feeling begins to emanate from your solar plexus produces distinct and ever increasing sensations of discomfort, it is important that as soon as you begin to notice this discomfort, you stop eating immediately, no matter how much or how little food is left on your plate.

When I teach this on my seminars, there is invariably one person who starts to panic and say, 'But what if I'm hungry again ten minutes later?'

The answer is very simple: if you're hungry, EAT. However, you must eat what you actually want, not what you think you should; eat CONSCIOUSLY and enjoy every mouthful, and then when you even suspect you are full, STOP.

REVISITING THE HUNGER SCALE

If you have been a serial dieter, you may be so used to overriding your body's signals that you keep eating until you're full or even stuffed before noticing it's time to stop. I cannot overemphasize what a useful tool the hunger scale will be for you. Becoming aware of what your body needs and wants is like a muscle – the more you use your awareness, the stronger it gets. When it comes to knowing when enough is enough, you'll want to stop eating at around 6 or 7 on the hunger scale – when you are feeling pleasantly satisfied or full but not yet stuffed or bloated. Simply, **never** live in the extreme areas of the hunger scale ever again.

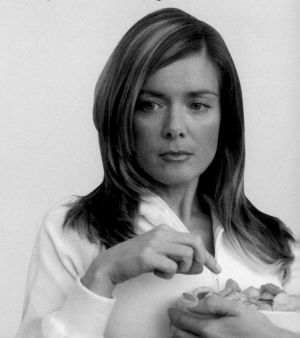

THE HUNGER SCALE

1. **Physically faint**

2. **Ravenous**

3. **Fairly hungry**

4. **Slightly hungry**

5. **Neutral**

6. **Pleasantly satisfied**

7. **Full**

8. **Stuffed**

9. **Bloated**

10. **Nauseous**

RESETTING THE THERMOSTAT

Here's a simple exercise I teach on my live seminars you may find useful to do for yourself.

1. Stop for a moment and remember a time when you were really hungry, or even starving. What did it feel like? Where in your body did you feel it? Really remember it in every detail now.

2. Next, remember a time when you felt completely stuffed. What did that feel like? Where in your body did you feel it? Again, remind yourself exactly what that felt like now.

3. When you're ready, compare the difference between the two feelings. What's it like to feel really hungry? What's it like to feel stuffed? Keep going back and forth between the two extremes about ten times to help your body to remember and recalibrate.

It may not feel like much is happening when you first do this exercise, but your body and unconscious mind are beginning an important process of recalibrating your inner signals. Each time you repeat it, it becomes easier to notice when you are truly hungry and stop eating as soon as you are full.

CHANGING THE HABITS OF A LIFETIME

I was with a friend of mine recently who had been a serial dieter but only seemed to be getting a little bit fatter and a lot more frustrated each year. In less than six months, he has lost four stone using this system. At first he wasn't sure if it was working, but he stuck to it and after a couple of weeks he noticed his clothes felt looser. He hadn't even done any of the mind-programming techniques – I had simply taught him the four golden rules that I have just taught you and he started using them.

When we were at dinner he only ate about half of his meal – a delicious-looking plate of pasta in a rich, creamy sauce. When I asked him if there was anything wrong with his food, he replied, 'No – it's delicious. But ever since you taught me that bloody system, I can't seem to overeat any more.'

He told me that he didn't even have to think about applying it – it had become second nature to him in a matter of weeks. This is typical of the progression most people experience. In the beginning, you need to consciously learn and apply each step. Then it begins to get easier and easier, and before you know it, you just do it because it's natural – the way your body was designed to eat.

When it comes to losing weight and keeping it off, habit is most people's worst enemy. For you, it will be different. We're going to recondition your habits and make them work for you. The mind-programming techniques throughout this book and on the CD will reinforce those new habits as the changes begin happening almost immediately.

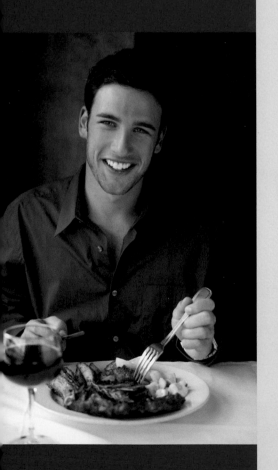

RESIGNING FROM THE 'CLEAN PLATE CLUB'

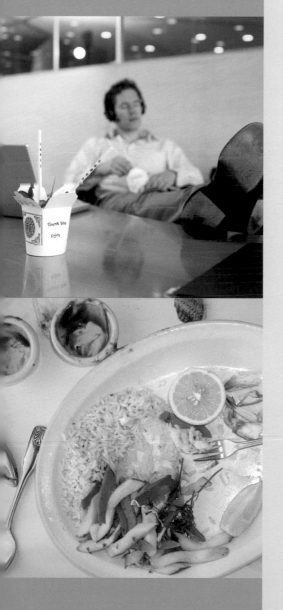

Why would anyone eat if they weren't hungry?

One of Professor Wansink's experiments involved drilling two holes in the bottom of a table at a university restaurant and placing two bowls with attached tubes over the holes. The plan was that he would be able to secretly refill the bowls without the diners noticing. On the opposite side of the table, he set two ordinary bowls.

When the students came into the cafeteria, he told them that he was conducting an experiment into the quality of the soup. In reality, the exact same soup was served to everyone. The difference was that the diners eating from the bowls with the holes in them didn't notice that, as they ate the soup, their bowls were being gradually refilled. Instead of listening to the signal from their stomach that said they had enough, they just kept on eating until they finished what was in the bowl. The result was that on average they ate a whopping 73 per cent more than the other diners.

One of the main habits that gets in the way of listening to your body is being a lifetime member of what I call the 'Clean Plate Club'. Members of this 'club' think that unless they finish everything put in front of them, they are somehow misbehaving.

But eating everything on your plate whether you're still hungry and enjoying it or not is basically giving permission for your weight to be controlled by some kid in a fast-food joint. Let's face it, you wouldn't let a shop assistant tell you how much to spend on clothes, would you?

Like most kids, I was told by my parents to eat everything on my plate because 'there are starving children in India'. Don't underestimate the subtle power of this guilt trip, especially if it was installed at a formative age. Eventually, of course, I realized that it was a con. I used to say, 'How does me being overweight help the starving children? Shall I take a picture of myself fat and send it to them with a note saying, "At least you know the food isn't going to waste?"'

Let me put this one to rest once and for all – contrary to popular parental opinion, eating everything on your plate has been shown to do nothing to contribute to the wellbeing of starving children in Africa, India or China. If you really want to play your part in putting an end to world hunger, learn to manage your eating so that you eat when you're hungry, enjoy every mouthful and stop when you think you're full. You'll wind up eating so much less that there'll be more for everyone else.

Of course, some members of the Clean Plate Club aren't so concerned about world hunger – they feel guilty leaving a half-eaten chicken breast on their plate. But no matter how hard you try to resuscitate the other half of the chicken breast, it isn't coming back to life. Now, I don't know about you, but I find it difficult to imagine a chicken sitting up in chicken heaven looking down on you in judgement should you leave part of its body on your plate.

Another popular excuse I hear from people is that it would be insulting to the chef if they leave any food uneaten. For this one, I find the easiest thing is to blame me. Just tell them you used my mind-programming CD and that while you would love to eat the extra six portions of mashed potatoes in gravy, I have somehow messed with your mind and you can now only eat half as much as you used to.

One of the simplest ways to give up your membership of the Clean Plate Club for good is simply to deliberately leave a bit of food on your plate, even if it's just one little chip. In this way, you are sending a new message to your unconscious mind, letting it know for sure that you are changing. Once you've broken the spell (by leaving a little food on your plate each time you eat), you'll feel comfortable eating only until you feel full, even if it means leaving half the food on your plate or more. You'll have less food in your stomach and more control in your life.

(And if you get hungry again later, not to worry – get another plate and leave some food on that one as well!)

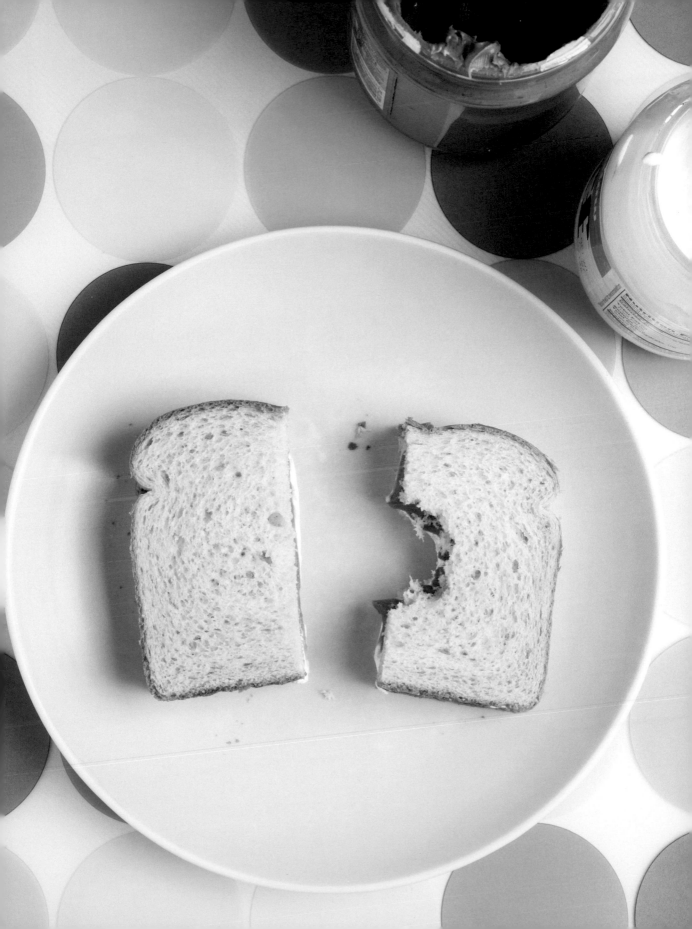

THE MAGIC WEIGHT-LOSS ELIXIR

There is one other thing that will support you in your efforts to eat only when you are hungry and stop as soon as you even suspect you are full.

Our bodies are made up of roughly 75 per cent water, and that percentage increases to nearly 85 per cent in the all-important area of brain tissue. When the inner mechanism in our body that regulates water levels senses any sort of a current or impending shortage, your body goes into selective water rationing mode. The brain gets first call on the water supply, with each internal organ receiving just enough water to maintain basic functioning.

According to Dr F. Batmanghelidj, author of the ground-breaking work **Your Body's Many Cries for Water**, many of the aches and pains that people experience on a daily basis, including hunger, are actually the preliminary effects of dehydration. This is one of the reasons why sometimes no matter what you eat, it doesn't feel as though it 'hits the spot'.

Because it's virtually impossible to tell the difference between this 'thirst signal' and authentic hunger, it's a good idea to make your first response to hunger pangs a fresh glass of water. If you're not hungry afterwards, it was thirst; if you still are, dig in!

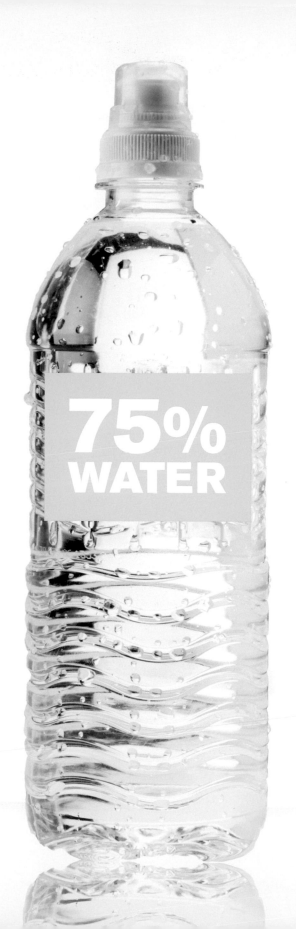

1

IT WILL FEEL A LITTLE WEIRD

WHAT TO EXPECT IN THE NEXT TWO WEEKS

Some people tell me that at first they felt a little bit self-conscious eating slowly and consciously chewing each mouthful, as though other people were staring at them. As the saying goes: 'You would worry less about what other people thought of you if you knew how seldom they did.' Most people are so caught up in their own heads they don't even notice what's going into their mouths, let alone what's going on with yours.

Also, people who know you as a serial dieter may notice the pizza, bacon and chocolate on your plate and smirk, thinking that you've 'fallen off another diet'.

This time, the last laugh will be on them. As it becomes easier and easier to eat consciously, your food will taste better and better and you will enjoy the wonderful feeling of satisfaction that comes from being in control of your eating.

In a society as filled with mixed messages about eating and body image as ours, what is considered 'normal' may be a long way from what is actually natural. While it may feel a bit odd at first to reprogram your body to eat in a new, more intuitive way, it is important to recognize you are actually moving towards a more natural way of eating. This is why it is sustainable – unlike diets, which go against your natural urge to eat when you are hungry and stop when you are full, the simplest weight-loss system in the world works with your body.

2

YOU WILL FEEL GOOD

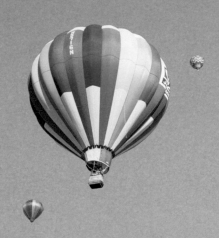

One of the most consistent benefits people report from using the simplest weight-loss system in the world is that they feel better – better in their bodies and better in themselves.

Here's what to expect:

- For the first time in ages you will feel more in control around food.

- The pressure of worrying about what to eat and when will be gone. It will be liberating to know you are free from the slavery of obsessing about food.

- You will see that it truly is possible for you to lose weight easily.

- You will realize that slim people are not different to you. We are all the same in our ability to lose weight.

In fact, you will be amazed at how easy it is!

Because you are not spending so much energy worrying about food, you will have more energy available for your life. This extra energy is one of the signs that the system is working perfectly.

3

YOU WILL WONDER HOW WELL IT'S WORKING

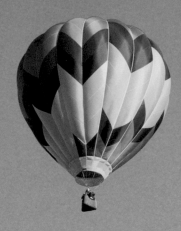

People who have successfully used this system often say that within the first couple of weeks they weren't sure if it was working. Whether you feel like you are eating more than before, or that you're not eating nutritionally balanced meals, or even like nothing much is different . . .

Relax!

As long as you are following the four golden rules, it's working.

It's normal to have doubts simply because you are doing something very different from what you have done before. Soon, as you begin to notice increased levels of energy, a slight change in how your clothes fit and a general sense of wellbeing in your body, you will realize that everything is working perfectly. Remember, you have already tried all sorts of other systems, diets or techniques and they haven't worked, or they've only worked for a short time. By committing to my system for the next two weeks, you've got nothing to lose except weight.

4

YOU WILL AT SOME POINT FORGET TO FOLLOW MY INSTRUCTIONS AND BREAK AT LEAST ONE IF NOT ALL FOUR OF THE GOLDEN RULES

It's important for you to know that YOU WILL have a slip or two along the way, shoving in a sandwich on the run, gorging yourself on chocolate digestives, eating to calm your nerves or even a full-on binge.

At this point you have a choice:

You can beat yourself up (like you've done in the past) and give up, telling yourself that you're a worthless piece of shit and you're never going to change.

Or:

You can RELAX, smile, remind yourself that I told you this would happen, and return to eating what you want when you are hungry, consciously enjoying each mouthful and stopping when you think you are full. No matter what happens, always go back to following my instructions. Give this system a fair go and you'll be glad of it for the rest of your life . . .

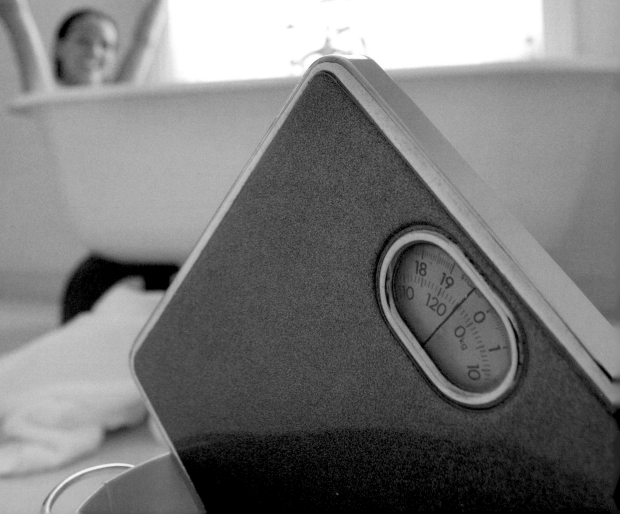

GET READY
TO GIVE UP
THE SCALES
FOR LIFE

WEIGHING YOURSELF

Let me offer you one final note of caution. Over the years that I have been working with weight-loss clients, I have noticed how many people are absolutely obsessed with weighing themselves. Some do it every day; some even do it after every meal, treating the scales like the lottery, expecting to see that suddenly they have lost a couple of stone since lunchtime.

**You cannot get an accurate reading on
your weight loss by checking every day.**

Each time you climb on to those scales, all you are doing is setting yourself up to feel bad. Everybody's weight goes up and down all the time – even slim people. In fact, naturally thin people rarely if ever weigh themselves. Most of them couldn't tell you what they weigh if you paid them.

Because weight can fluctuate by as much as ten pounds up or down from environmental factors, water retention and even atmospheric pressure, it is actually the least reliable measure on the road to becoming thin. So it is important that you DO NOT WEIGH YOURSELF for the next two weeks.

I recommend that you give up the scales for life – you'll know you're thin because you look great and you feel wonderful. However, if you absolutely must weigh yourself, leave at least TWO weeks between each weighing.

When an aeroplane flies from one place to another it doesn't fly in a straight line – it's always adjusting its course. Despite the fact that it's off course as much as 91 per cent of the time, it always knows where it's going.

It's the same with losing weight – while some days will be better than others and sometimes you will feel more confident about your weight than others, if you keep your eye on the prize and keep following the guidelines, YOU WILL LOSE WEIGHT and keep it off, for as long as you use this system.

CAN IT REALLY BE THIS SIMPLE?

YES! LET'S REVIEW THE FOUR ELEMENTS OF THE SYSTEM:

1 **Eat when you're hungry.**

2 **Eat only what you want, never what you think you 'should'.**

3 **Eat consciously and enjoy every mouthful.**

4 **Stop when you even think you're full.**

That is all you need to do in order to lose weight and keep it off for life. And if you're truly ready to be thin, I can make it even simpler for you. If you change only one thing about the way that you eat, do this:

CONSCIOUSLY ENJOY EVERY MOUTHFUL

By focusing on this one element of the system, everything else will fall into place, because:

- You can't and won't get the full enjoyment out of your food if you're not properly hungry.

- You can only truly enjoy your food when you choose only foods you truly enjoy.

- Your food will stop being enjoyable if you don't stop eating when your body is full.

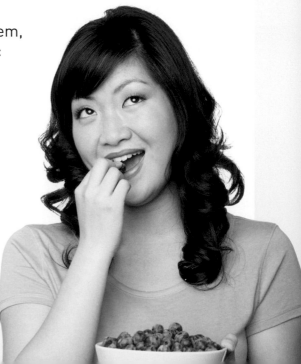

LOOK GREAT
FEEL WONDERFUL

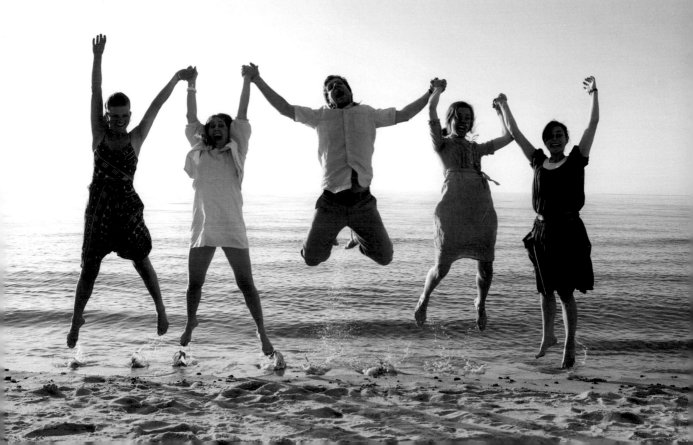

CLAIRE SINGH

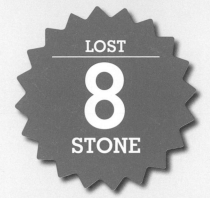

LOST

8

STONE

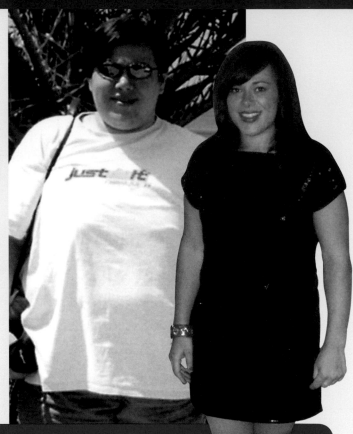

CLAIRE'S STORY

My weight had been a problem for most of my adult life. If you'd asked me what I ate in a day, I'd have told you, and it might not have sounded much. But that's because I wasn't even registering what I was eating.

My mum paid for Paul's workshop as a present. I decided to go since I had nothing to lose. I'll never forget that day. It was such a huge revelation, as if someone had just woken me up and said, 'Here are the answers.'

I now view food in a completely different way. Food is fuel for the body, not a life crutch. Ever since attending Paul's workshop, I've eaten a lot less. I think about what I eat and become full more easily. I don't eat junk food, and I've improved my cooking skills. As well as being thinner, I'm more in tune with my body now, and no longer suffer from a poor digestive system. It's like someone said, 'Here's a key to the rest of your life . . .'

My top tip: I still listen to Paul's CD. It's useful for refocusing my mind, and it's supportive.

FREQUENTLY ASKED QUESTIONS ABOUT 'THE SIMPLEST WEIGHT-LOSS SYSTEM IN THE WORLD'

Q. What if I can't tell when I am full?

In his book **Achieving Vibrance**, Gay Hendricks teaches about a mechanism in the body he calls 'the V spot', which is located in your solar plexus, just below your ribcage and towards the centre of your body. This is actually a muscle designed to control the flow of food to the stomach. Unfortunately, it's not a very strong muscle for most of us. However, as you get more and more sensitive to your body's signals, you can actually feel the V spot close off when your body has had enough food.

In the meantime, just stop if you suspect you might be full, knowing that it doesn't matter if you're wrong – you can always start eating again if it turns out your body is still hungry.

Q. It's a huge relief to eat when I'm hungry, but I feel guilty eating whatever I want. Can I do one without the other?

No, no, no, no and no. One of the worst consequences of the diet conspiracy is that serial dieters are continually looking over their shoulder for the food police, lest they be caught enjoying food and sent back to starvation purgatory. Your body was made to run on food, and it will always tell you what it needs once you learn to listen.

Every time you eat something you don't really want, you're reinforcing the idea that someone other than you and your body knows best about what you need – and while that's great news for the advertising industry, it's a recipe for disaster when it comes to losing weight.

Chapter
Three

PROGRAM YOUR MIND TO SLIM YOUR BODY

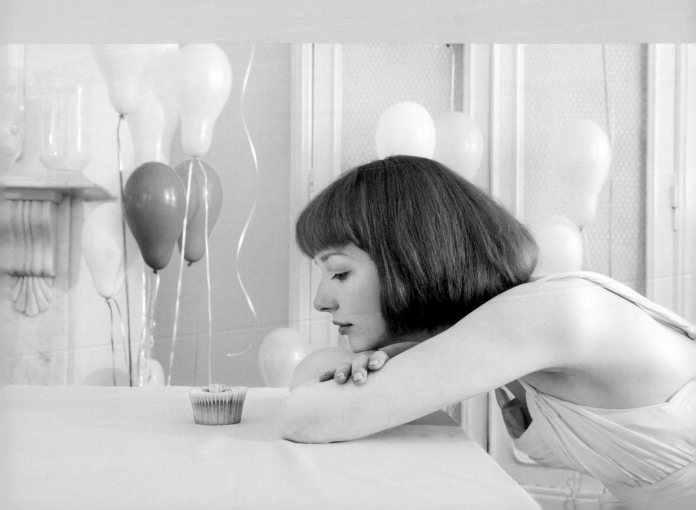

THE HABITS OF A LIFETIME

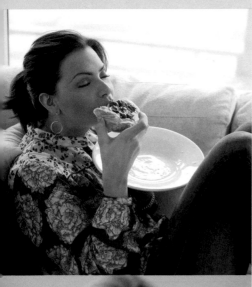

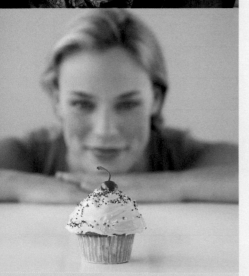

I know there have been many times in the past when you've done your best to eat sensibly, but no matter how hard you tried, you couldn't stick with it. And you probably thought that in some way it was your fault – if only you had more willpower, you wouldn't be overweight.

Based on the latest scientific data, I can address that issue once and for all:

Rubbish!

The truth is that it's nearly impossible to break a habit with willpower alone – you have to reprogram your mind. With the right programs in place, doing the right thing is easy; with the wrong programs running your mind, it's virtually impossible.

Over the years, I have helped people change life-long compulsions in a matter of minutes and proved that even the most die-hard addiction will succumb to effective reprogramming. Yet until you've experienced it for yourself, this may seem a bit different. After all, if lasting changes can happen this quickly and this easily, why haven't you been able to do it in the past?

It all boils down to a simple psychological rule:

**Your imagination is far
more powerful than your will.**

To give yourself a quick experience of this, imagine a piece of chocolate cake (or your favourite food) in front of you. Next, tell yourself with all your willpower that you are not going to eat it. Then imagine the taste of that chocolatey icing as it melts on your tongue. Can you feel your will weakening yet?

Next, once again imagine that piece of chocolate cake (or your favourite food) in front of you. Now, imagine the cake is covered in maggots – slimy, wriggling maggots. Notice the foul smell emanating from the maggots (or is it the cake?). Has the cake lost some of its appeal?

That's the power of your imagination in action. In fact, it's through your imagination that you actually make all your best decisions about what you are going to eat. When you read the menu in a restaurant, you mentally taste all the food in your mind before you decide what to have. That's why restaurants go to such trouble to describe their food in appetizing terms. For example, which would you rather have for dinner this evening: 'Goujons of sole lightly sautéed and served in a delicate lemon sauce' or 'Dead fish'?

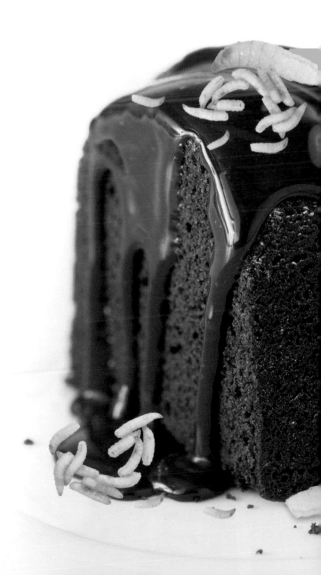

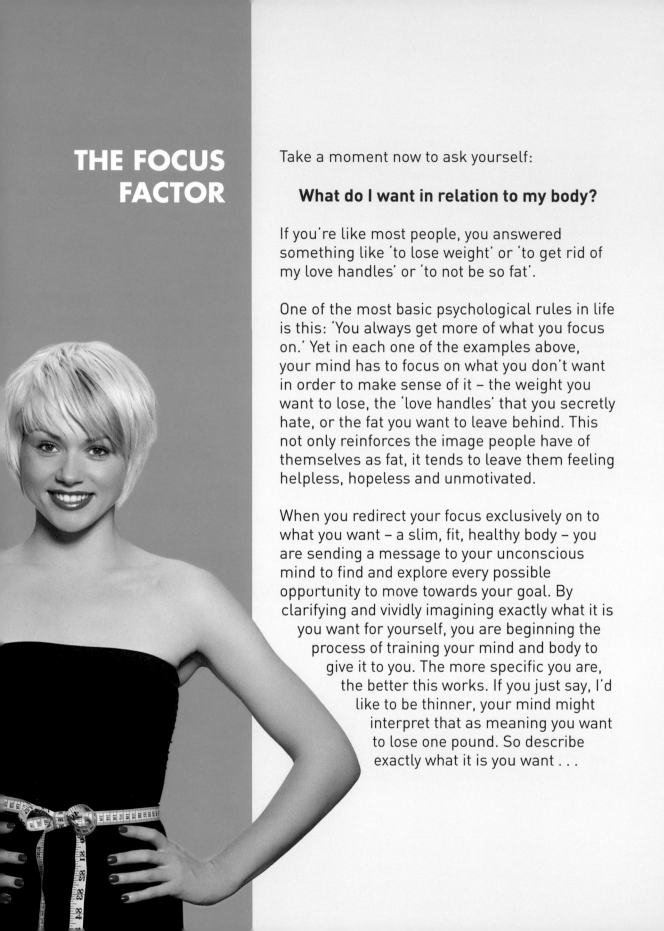

THE FOCUS FACTOR

Take a moment now to ask yourself:

What do I want in relation to my body?

If you're like most people, you answered something like 'to lose weight' or 'to get rid of my love handles' or 'to not be so fat'.

One of the most basic psychological rules in life is this: 'You always get more of what you focus on.' Yet in each one of the examples above, your mind has to focus on what you don't want in order to make sense of it – the weight you want to lose, the 'love handles' that you secretly hate, or the fat you want to leave behind. This not only reinforces the image people have of themselves as fat, it tends to leave them feeling helpless, hopeless and unmotivated.

When you redirect your focus exclusively on to what you want – a slim, fit, healthy body – you are sending a message to your unconscious mind to find and explore every possible opportunity to move towards your goal. By clarifying and vividly imagining exactly what it is you want for yourself, you are beginning the process of training your mind and body to give it to you. The more specific you are, the better this works. If you just say, I'd like to be thinner, your mind might interpret that as meaning you want to lose one pound. So describe exactly what it is you want . . .

For example:

I WANT TO LOSE FOUR STONE IN THE NEXT FOUR MONTHS.

Or:

I WANT TO FEEL COMFORTABLE IN A SIZE-12 DRESS.

Or my personal favourite:

I WANT TO LOOK GREAT NAKED!

SELF IMAGE AND THE SELF FULFILLING PROPHECY

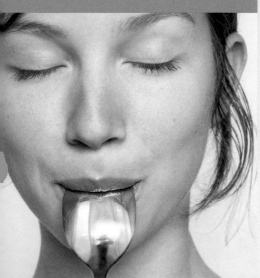

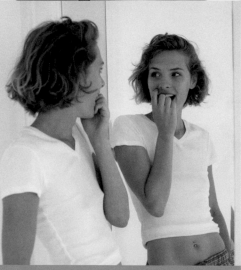

Remember, all you need to do to reach your goal is:

1. Eat when you're hungry.

2. Eat what you actually want.

3. Eat consciously and enjoy every mouthful.

4. Stop when you think you're full.

So why keep reading?

Because the techniques that follow will make the whole process happen even more easily and allow you to feel significantly better about yourself as well. In other words:

**We are not only what we eat,
but what we think as well.**

In the 1960s the famous plastic surgeon Maxwell Maltz found that after many of his operations, the self-esteem and confidence levels of his patients rose dramatically. However, for a few people the operations didn't seem to make any difference. After a great deal of exploration, Dr Maltz concluded that those patients who didn't experience a change in their levels of wellbeing were 'scarred on the inside'. They saw themselves as unworthy, bad or hopeless, and the fact that their appearance had changed on the outside made no difference to the image they held of themselves on the inside. They had what he called 'an impoverished self-image'.

Your self-image is how you see yourself in your imagination. It's the blueprint that determines everything about you, from how motivated, intelligent and confident you are willing to let yourself be, to how much weight you are willing to carry around with you or lose.

The reason our self-image has such a powerful influence on our behaviour is that it is self-reinforcing. For example, we've all met people who are not classically good-looking but have an aura of attractiveness. Because they think of themselves as attractive, they carry themselves well, dress to bring out their most attractive features, and have the confidence to speak to anyone. This self-confidence makes them attractive to others, who respond positively to them, which reinforces their image of themselves as attractive.

Equally, there are plenty of people who think of themselves as unattractive, and unconsciously sabotage any attempts to appear attractive. After all, if you truly believe you are unattractive, why take the time to dress mutton up as lamb? However, if you don't do what it takes to represent yourself at your best, people will inevitably find you unattractive.

Either way, your self-image has worked perfectly, 'proving' itself right by guiding you to act consistently with who you believe yourself to be.

Nearly every overweight person has a self-image that says they will always be fat. While they may say they would prefer to be thin, they often think that thin people are somehow different from them, and the goal seems almost unattainable.

How do you change the pattern?

By getting into the habit of focusing your attention on what you DO want. Like it or not, you're going to need to get used to thinking of yourself with an attractive body!

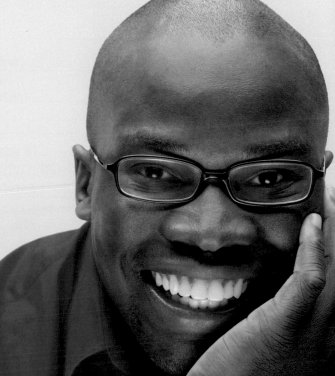

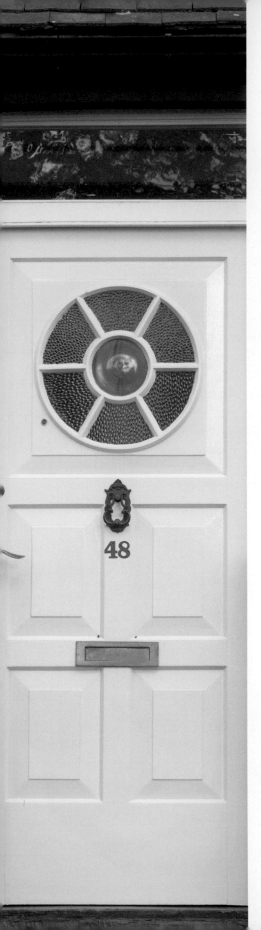

SEE YOURSELF SLIM

Recent scientific research in the United States and Europe has conclusively shown that visualization techniques dramatically enhance your ability to lose weight. As you vividly imagine yourself slim and rehearse your path to your ideal weight, you send a message to your brain that affects your energy levels, your motivation and your metabolism. Those changes cause physical sensations, which in turn affect your thoughts and emotions, which in turn reinforce the programming you are giving your brain. It's a positive feedback system, and every element of the system gets to feel good as you lose weight.

As I guide you through these next two exercises, I am going to be instructing you to visualize. This is something everyone already has the ability to do. To prove this to yourself, answer the following questions:

1. **What does your front door look like?**

2. **What colour is it?**

3. **Which side is the handle on?**

In order to answer any of these questions, you had to visualize – to go into your imagination and make pictures. Now, for 99 per cent of people, these mental images will not be as real as reality – and that's a good thing. People who can't tell the difference between the pictures in their head and what they see in the world are in trouble.

YOUR PERFECT BODY

Here's a simple but powerful exercise that will train your unconscious mind to help you lose weight and keep it off. Before you do this exercise, read through all the steps first.

1 Stop for a moment and imagine you are watching a movie of a thin, happy, confident you.

2 Watch that thinner you doing the things you do in your daily life and accomplishing them with ease. Imagine this new you eating just the right amount, moving their body regularly, and handling their emotional needs quickly and easily.

- How does that other you talk to themselves?
- What kind of voice tone do they use?
- How do they carry themselves?
- How do they move?

3 If the movie is not yet exactly how you want things to be, make the adjustments that make you feel great. Allow your intuition to be your guide.

4 When you are satisfied with the other you, step into it. Take the new perspective and behaviours into you.

5 Now run the movie and imagine being in all of your daily situations and view them from your new perspective. Think through what it's like to have this new perspective and what it will help you to achieve. How are things going to be so much better now?

REPETITION
REPETITION
REPETITION

Remember, repetition is the key to success. When we repeat an action, a neural pathway is created in the brain and each repetition reinforces it. As you think of yourself as slim and healthy you are sending signals to your unconscious mind to behave, to feel and to eat like a slim person. As your body gets lighter you will feel more sensitive, more energetic and more alive.

Do the Perfect Body exercise (on the previous page) every morning and, before long, it will become a healthy habit. The more you do this the sooner you will start to feel better and change the way you feel about yourself for the better. Each time you do it, you will be one step closer to your ideal weight.

This exercise focuses your mind on your target, making it more powerful and more and more compelling, so that every time you say no to the foods you no longer wish to eat and yes to those foods you do want, you will feel more of this delightful lightness and know you are one step closer to your ideal weight.

In addition, each time you listen to the special mind-programming CD, you will be reinforcing all the gains you make each time you take the time to see yourself slim.

I CAN MAKE YOU

THIN

PA
McK
Record
by M

FREQUENTLY ASKED QUESTIONS ABOUT 'PROGRAM YOUR MIND TO SLIM YOUR BODY'

Q. What do I do if I'm having trouble seeing myself in my mind's eye?

Just keep listening to the CD and let me do the work. You wouldn't go to a restaurant and expect to cook your own dinner, would you? All you need to do is sit back, relax and let the powerful suggestions on the mind-programming CD do their job. By the time you've listened at least once a day for at least two weeks, your mind and body will have already begun to change for the better.

Q. I find that I fall asleep listening to the CD. Will it still work for me?

Yes – in some ways it will work even more easily than when you stay awake and listen consciously!

Any new mother knows that no matter how deeply she sleeps with one part of her mind, another part of her mind will wake her up immediately if her baby starts to cry.

Similarly, even while your body sleeps, your unconscious mind is listening. All the positive messages from the CD are going directly into your unconscious, reinforcing your new, healthy relationship with food each and every time you listen. As an additional resource, I have created an online club at www.mckenna.com where you can get complete support in losing weight and keeping it off for life. As a member, you'll be able to watch mini-movies demonstrating each of the techniques featured in this book and receive coaching from me and others who have successfully lost weight and kept it off using this system. Please note, becoming a member is not necessary in order for you to succeed; however, many people have reported how much they appreciate being part of a community of like-minded people as they move forward with their own weight-loss goals.

Q. I can't seem to quit the Clean Plate Club no matter how hard I try – do you have any further suggestions?

It sounds as though you are still trying to 'willpower' yourself thin, which is a bit like trying to hammer in nails with nothing but a screwdriver. It's not that it's not a useful tool, but rather that it's the wrong tool for the job at hand. By using your imagination instead of your will, you'll find it nearly effortless to leave food on your plate and out of your stomach.

If you're really stuck, try this – cut off a few bites of food before you start eating and either throw them away or sweep them onto a spare plate and have your waiter or waitress take it away. Then you can eat everything that's left on your plate (providing you're actually hungry).

If after all that you still find yourself feeling guilty about leaving that half-eaten chicken breast or nut cutlet on your plate, you can use the tapping technique that I will share with you in Chapter Six to eliminate the unnecessary guilt and move on with your healthy body and healthier life.

AMANDA SAMSON

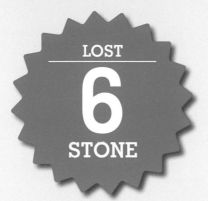

LOST

6

STONE

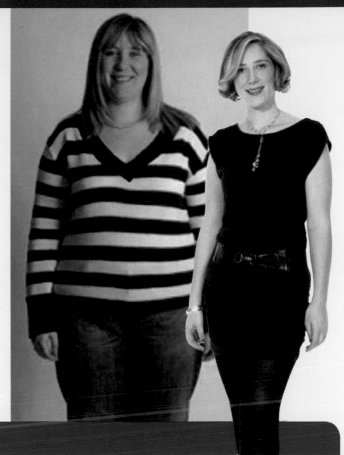

AMANDA'S STORY

My life was miserable, my diet was miserable and I was miserable. Now, 6 stone lighter, I have a new lease of life.

I wasn't sure, after years of dieting, that this would work. Nothing else did. So I set out with low expectations – and two weeks later I had lost 9 pounds! All I did was follow the four golden rules. I kept on eating all my favourite foods, and nobody even knew I was trying to lose weight.

To begin with, I struggled with knowing when I was hungry, so at first I just guessed, and after listening to my body for a while it got easier and easier. Before I knew it, my new eating habits had become a way of life. I could never go back to eating the way I used to. My life is now happy, my diet is now happy and I am happy – what more could you want!

My top tip: EAT CONSCIOUSLY was the part of the system that worked best for me.

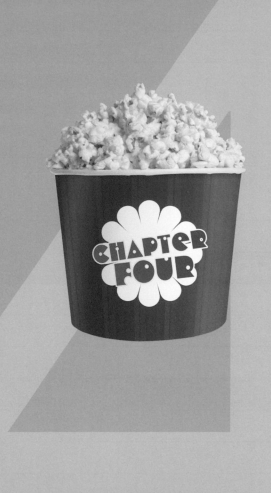

CHAPTER FOUR

OVERCOMING EMOTIONAL EATING

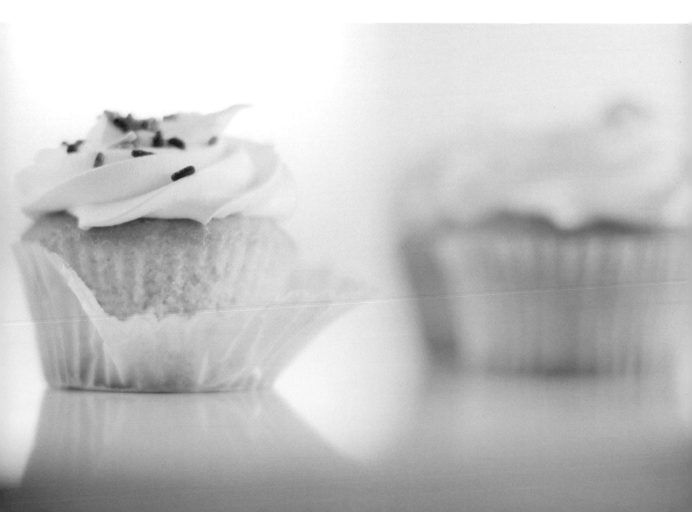

RECOGNIZING EMOTIONAL HUNGER

> *IT'S AMAZING. I CAN HONESTLY SAY I HAVEN'T EATEN CHOCOLATE SINCE I STARTED USING PAUL'S SYSTEM. PRIOR TO THAT I WAS EATING TEN BARS A DAY!*
>
> GILL MITCHELL, SOCIAL WORKER

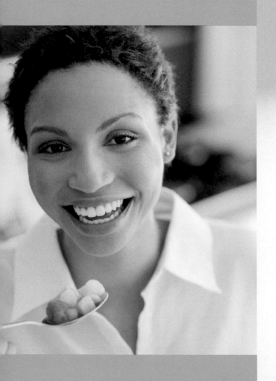

One of the most common mistakes people make when they first start out on my system is to confuse emotional hunger with physical hunger. This is because until we become more attuned to our bodies, the two feel remarkably similar.

In fact, the number-one reason people eat when they're not hungry is to cover up a negative emotion or to fill an emotional hole. That's why you can sometimes find yourself eating and eating without getting full – you were never hungry for food in the first place.

Perhaps you had an argument and had some chocolate to make yourself feel better, or you got home after a long, hard day and decided to cheer yourself up with some ice cream. Maybe you just were feeling bored and suddenly decided that a plate of cheese and crackers would hit the spot. But as my friend Michael Neill says, 'There aren't enough cookies in the world to make you feel loved and whole.'

Here are a couple of pointers to help you make a clear distinction every time:

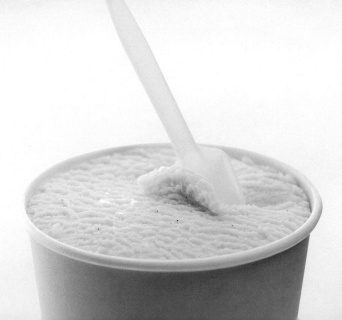

1 EMOTIONAL HUNGER IS SUDDEN AND URGENT; PHYSICAL HUNGER IS GRADUAL AND PATIENT

Have you ever had the experience of having a sudden, desperate craving for food?

If you track back in your mind, you'll find that only moments before the 'hunger' arrived, you were having an argument with yourself in your mind. In order to not deal with whatever feelings are going on in your body, people learn to bury those feelings with food.

Physical hunger, on the other hand, is gradual. You may notice a gentle griping in your tummy, or even a deep rumbling. If you continue to ignore your hunger, you'll probably experience light-headedness or even sadness, anger and tiredness. The earlier you learn to pick up on your body's 'hints' that it needs fuel, the easier it will be to separate out these two signals.

2 EMOTIONAL HUNGER CANNOT BE SATISFIED WITH FOOD; PHYSICAL HUNGER CAN

If you are eating and eating and never feeling satisfied, it's because you don't need food – you need to change your feelings. When you're hungry for good feelings (or at least a temporary masking of bad feelings), no amount of food will do the trick. This is an additional way in which emotional hunger differs from physical hunger – when you address the root cause of emotional hunger, it doesn't come back again four hours later.

Regardless of its specific manifestations, the feelings that underlie emotional hunger invariably come down to just one thing:

Inescapable stress

According to the latest thinking among researchers into craving and addiction, 'inescapable stress' is the ongoing sense that nothing can be done to reduce the amount of stress you are experiencing in your life. That seemingly inescapable stress may take the form of a bad marriage or a chronic illness or even something as simple as stress at work. It can even be caused by guilt or shame – the regret for something that happened in the past that cannot be undone.

In his excellent book **The Craving Brain**, Dr Ronald Ruden points out that the experience of inescapable stress changes the landscape of the brain, creating a physiological craving for substances (such as food and/or alcohol) that will allow us to move our experience of stress into the background. In essence, food becomes a Band-aid that provides temporary relief without leading to any improvement in the situation that caused the stress in the first place.
Based on this cutting-edge research, we now have a 'magic pill' to help you lose weight:

**Control your response to stress,
and you will no longer want or need to overeat.**

As we have already learned, the mind and body are intimately linked. Recent scientific research has shown that our thoughts have a significant effect upon our health and wellbeing. We can change biological processes in the body through our imagination and we can certainly change our feelings and moods. As you reprogram your mind and develop your ability to respond to stress, you will actually change the neurochemical landscape of your brain.

In this next exercise, we are going to use a simple associational technique to create an inner sense of calm inside your body – the same sense of calm and peace you used to give yourself by overeating. By repeatedly doing this exercise and reinforcing it with the hypnotic suggestions on the CD, you will be able to lower your stress levels and gently eliminate your emotional hunger pangs without the worry, angst or struggle most people experience . . .

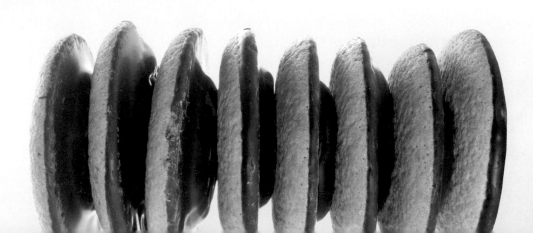

THE CALM ANCHOR

Before you do this exercise, read through all the steps first.

1. Remember a time when you felt really, really calm – at peace and in control. Fully return to it now, seeing what you saw, hearing what you heard and feeling how good you felt. (If you can't remember a time, imagine how wonderful it would feel to be totally at peace – if you had all the ease, comfort and self-control you could ever need.)

2. As you keep running through this experience in your mind, make the colours brighter and richer, the sounds crisper and the feelings stronger.

3. When you are feeling these good feelings, squeeze the thumb and middle finger of your right hand together. You are associating this particular pressure in this particular place with this particular emotion. Run through this memory several times until you feel a lovely sense of inner peace and calm.

4. Now go through this relaxing memory at least five more times while continuing to squeeze your thumb and middle finger together to really lock in these good feelings. You will know you have done it enough when all you need to do is squeeze your fingers together and you can easily remember the feelings of calm and relaxation spreading through your body.

5. Next, think about a situation that in the past you would have found mildly stressful. Once again, squeeze your thumb and middle finger together. Feel that calm feeling spreading through your body and imagine taking it with you into that stressful situation. Imagine everything going perfectly, exactly the way that you want. See what you'll see, hear what you hear and feel how good it feels to be so much calmer and in control in this situation.

6. Now, still squeezing your thumb and finger together, remember that calm feeling of being in control and once again imagine being in that situation that used to seem stressful. This time, imagine a few challenges occurring and notice yourself handling all the challenges perfectly. See what you'll see, hear what you hear and feel how good it feels to be so much calmer and in control in this situation.

Stop and think about that situation now. Notice the difference from only a few minutes ago. Do you feel less stressed and more in control? If not, just repeat the exercise until you do!

Each time you do this exercise, it will become easier and easier to experience feelings of relaxation at calm 'at your fingertips' . . .

YOUR HARSHEST CRITIC

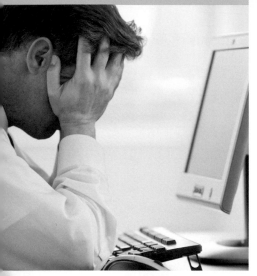

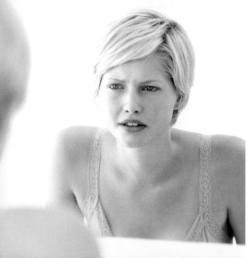

One of the most common sources of inescapable stress is a secret many people carry with them throughout their lives:

Self-loathing – feeling helpless, hopeless, worthless and unloved

I am continually amazed at the abuse most people subject themselves to at the start of each day. They'll look at themselves in the mirror in the morning, say 'fat face, fat arms, fat thighs, fat arse', and then go about their day wondering why they don't feel good about themselves.

On my weight-loss seminars I do an exercise where I help people stop the abuse and start to appreciate themselves. I ask for a volunteer to look into a mirror and share their internal criticism out loud with the group. Once, I was doing this exercise with a lovely-looking lady who saw herself in the mirror and immediately blurted out, 'Fat fucking cow.'

Of course, everyone burst out laughing because they could so easily identify with her. When I asked her what she would do if someone walked up to her in the street and said that to her, she replied that she would probably hit them. She wouldn't take it from someone else, but she'd readily insult herself every time she looked in the mirror.

Possibly the most famous guideline for effective living in western civilization is the so-called 'golden rule', which is generally expressed in some version of 'Do unto others as you would have done unto you'.

My candidate for a 'platinum rule' is this:

Do unto yourself as you would have others do unto you.

If anyone else insulted us as openly and crudely as we insult ourselves ('I'm such a stupid idiot', 'I'm so useless', 'I'm such a waste of space', 'God, I'm pathetic', etc.) or punished us as unforgivingly as we punish ourselves ('I can't believe I ate dessert – that's it! I'm going to work out until I throw up!'), we would be up in arms, protesting at the injustice and inhumanity of such cruel and unusual treatment.

But when we treat ourselves that way, we put up with it – mostly because nobody ever told us we didn't have to. Until you realize there are healthy alternatives to motivating yourself to lose weight by beating yourself up for being fat, you will find it virtually impossible to measure up to your own unrealistically high standards. Fortunately, by seeing self-loathing for what it is, you lessen its power over you and make it possible to address it directly instead of attempting to stuff it down with food.

As you begin to see yourself as capable, lovable and intrinsically worthy, you will continue to feel the

pangs of emotional hunger. When you are feeling low, it is commonplace that friends and family can see your strengths and value even when you do not. We can use this fact to begin the process of loving and valuing ourselves. Here's an exercise to help you begin to change the patterns of self-loathing that most of us have been carrying throughout our lives.

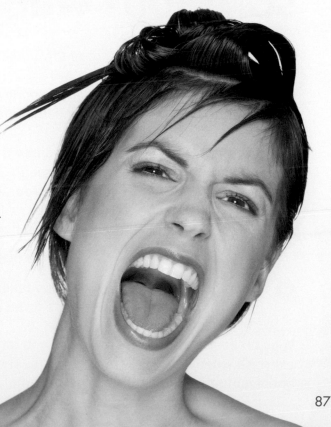

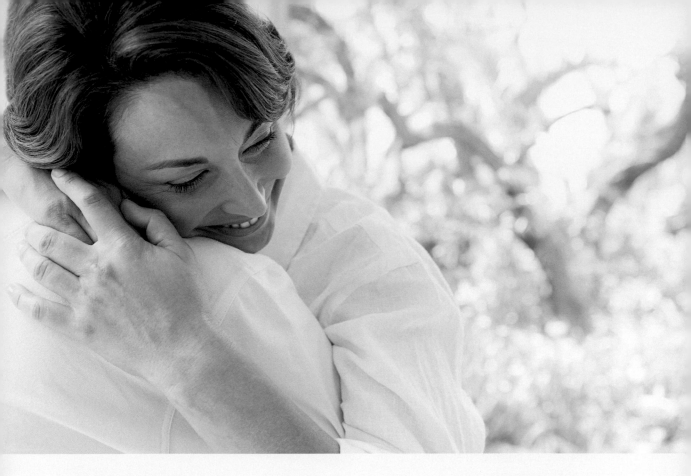

SOMEBODY WHO LOVES YOU

Before you do this exercise, read through all the steps first.

1 Close your eyes and think of someone who loves or deeply appreciates you. Remember how they look, and imagine they are standing in front of you now.

2 Gently step out of your body and into the body of the person who loves you. See through their eyes, hear through their ears, and feel the love and good feelings they have as you look at yourself. Really notice in detail what it is they love and appreciate about you. Recognize and acknowledge those amazing qualities that perhaps you hadn't appreciated about yourself until now.

3 Step back into your own body and take a few moments to enjoy those good feelings of knowing that you are loved and appreciated exactly as you are.

You can keep that inner feeling with you for hours and hours and rerun this exercise whenever you want to boost it. The more you do it, the easier it becomes, and eventually it becomes almost automatic to love and feel loved.

THE NATURAL DESIGN OF YOUR BODY

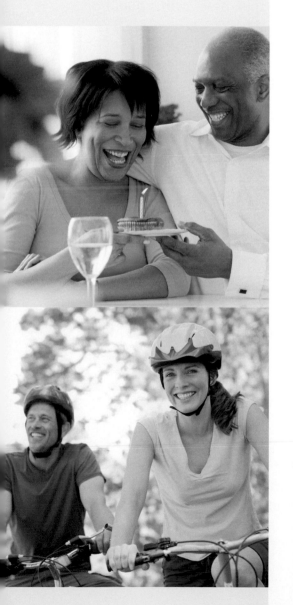

Did you know that less than one per cent of the women in the world even have the genetic potential for what is considered a 'model figure'? Yet when I meet people who consider themselves to be overweight, they spend an inordinate amount of time comparing themselves to airbrushed magazine images of smiling, anorexically thin women and make themselves feel so bad they need to eat something in order to feel better!

Our bodies contain a natural blueprint for optimal health. Human beings are designed to be around five or six feet tall, and that's why we stop growing in our late teens. No one carries on growing to twenty feet – it wouldn't be natural and it wouldn't be healthy. In the same way, we have a natural shape. If we get too much bigger or smaller than that, it's because we have interfered with the natural design of the body.

It is very common for people to tell me they don't like their body and will do whatever they can to try to ignore it. What they don't realize is that it is important to pay attention – if you want to change how you look, you must first make peace with your natural body. In fact, the more you learn to accept your body as it is, the more you'll be amazed at how effortlessly it changes.

Here's the bottom line:

You've got to make friends with the body you have in order to get the body you want.

Of course you may be looking forward to thinner thighs or a flatter tummy, but it is this same body you are already in that is going to be fitter and slimmer, so you may as well begin making peace with it now.

ANOREXIA, BULIMIA AND BODY DYSMORPHIA

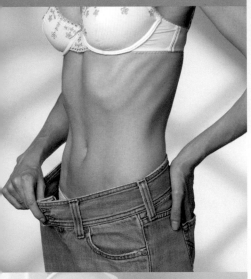

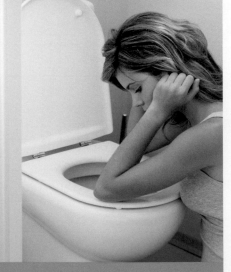

(All of the techniques in this book can make a real difference to the way you feel about yourself and the actions you take. In fact, many people with eating disorders have told me that the discipline of following this system and practising the self-esteem exercises has really helped them. However, if you suspect or have been told that you are suffering from an eating disorder, you should seek help from a qualified professional.)

Even though anorexics and bulimics are often painfully thin, they tell themselves how overweight they are and say all kinds of abusive things to themselves when they look in the mirror.

Some of them are able to telescope their vision on to some tiny aspect of themselves, focusing all their self-hate on to that one body part. Others are able to hallucinate, like looking in those fun-house mirrors at the seaside that make you appear much taller or wider than you really are. This distorted self-image, commonly referred to as body dysmorphia, keeps people from truly enjoying life or eating enough. At best it has dire health consequences; at worst it can be fatal.

I worked with a lovely-looking lady on TV who couldn't look at herself in the mirror without bursting into tears. She'd tried every kind of therapy and none of it had worked. Using the techniques that I am about to teach you, she overcame this horrible life-long disorder. In less than an hour, she was able to confidently look at herself in the mirror and see herself as beautiful.

During the change process I asked her to remember a time when she had been paid a compliment. Try as she might, she couldn't think of a single one.

Her partner was present and I suggested she think of a time when he'd said something nice to her. 'That'll be the day!' she said. He looked a little hurt and surprised and replied, 'I say nice things to you all the time.'

Before she had a chance to argue, I jumped in and said, 'I believe him!'

Our self-image acts as a filter for what fits with who we think we are. Because she had such a poor self-image, whenever anybody said anything nice to her she immediately dismissed it because it didn't fit with who she thought she was.

The sweetest moment in this session came at the end. Although she had been with her partner for several years and they had a child together, they had never got married because she couldn't bear the thought of 'all those people looking at me on my wedding day while I'm so hideous'.

After we had taken away the self-hate and she filled herself up with love, I asked her how she felt about getting married now. She turned, smiled at her partner and said, 'Well, someone will have to ask me.' She was finally able to let in all the love that he had been trying to give her for years.

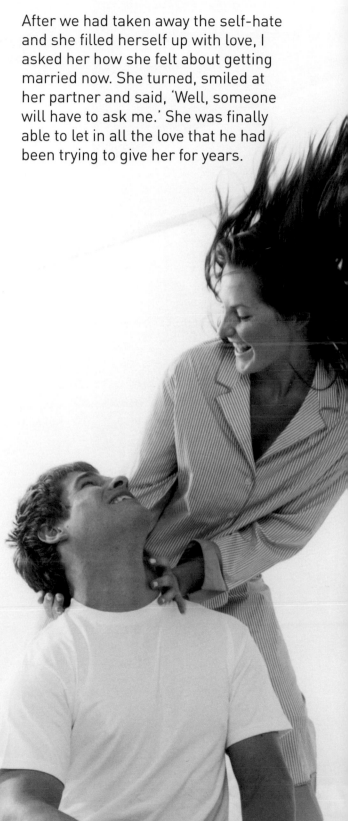

THE FRIENDLY MIRROR

Everyone receives compliments and praise from time to time. Sometimes they may seem trivial, like 'Hey, you're looking great' or 'You look sharp today'. At other times they may seem quite significant, like 'You are so sexy', or 'Do you know how much people respect you?'

Sincere, positive perceptions from others, which you might not have been able to see or fully appreciate from the point of view you had at the time, can be valuable in learning to appreciate your own qualities more fully and enhance your self-esteem now.

The next three techniques will help you to eliminate emotional hunger by enabling you to feel better and better about yourself every time you look in the mirror. Read through each technique several times until you know the steps and then go and do it. The entire process will take no more than ten minutes, and can be repeated as often as you choose.

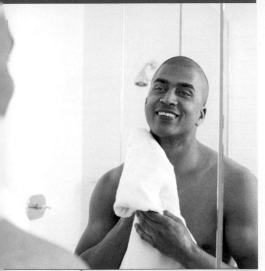

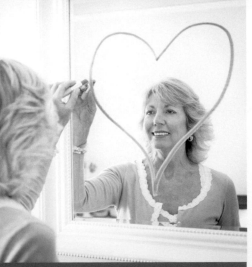

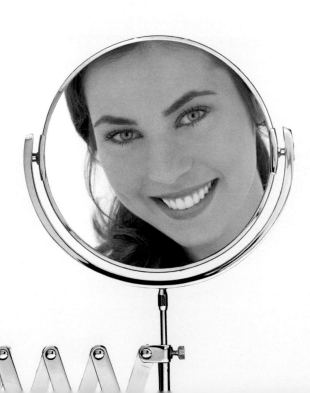

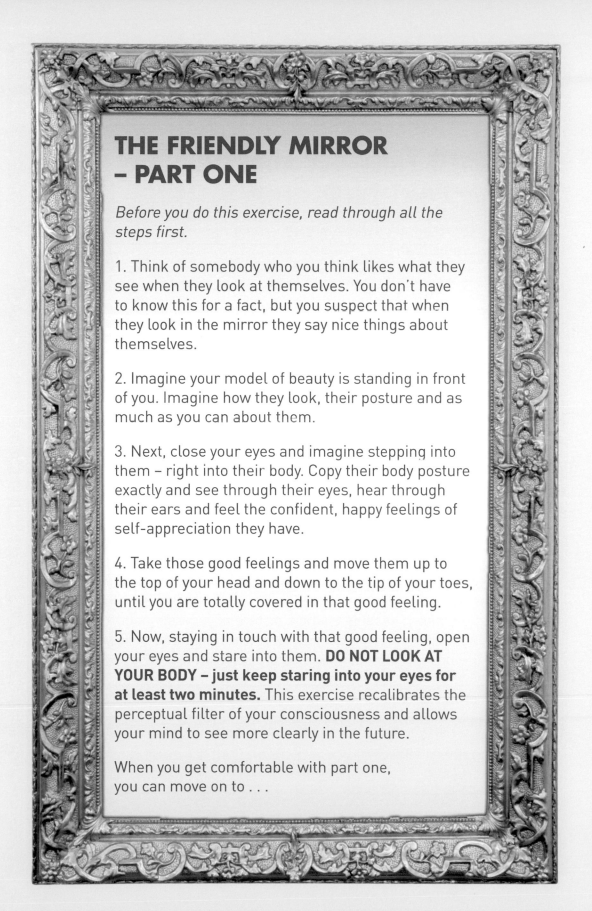

THE FRIENDLY MIRROR
– PART ONE

Before you do this exercise, read through all the steps first.

1. Think of somebody who you think likes what they see when they look at themselves. You don't have to know this for a fact, but you suspect that when they look in the mirror they say nice things about themselves.

2. Imagine your model of beauty is standing in front of you. Imagine how they look, their posture and as much as you can about them.

3. Next, close your eyes and imagine stepping into them – right into their body. Copy their body posture exactly and see through their eyes, hear through their ears and feel the confident, happy feelings of self-appreciation they have.

4. Take those good feelings and move them up to the top of your head and down to the tip of your toes, until you are totally covered in that good feeling.

5. Now, staying in touch with that good feeling, open your eyes and stare into them. **DO NOT LOOK AT YOUR BODY – just keep staring into your eyes for at least two minutes.** This exercise recalibrates the perceptual filter of your consciousness and allows your mind to see more clearly in the future.

When you get comfortable with part one,
you can move on to . . .

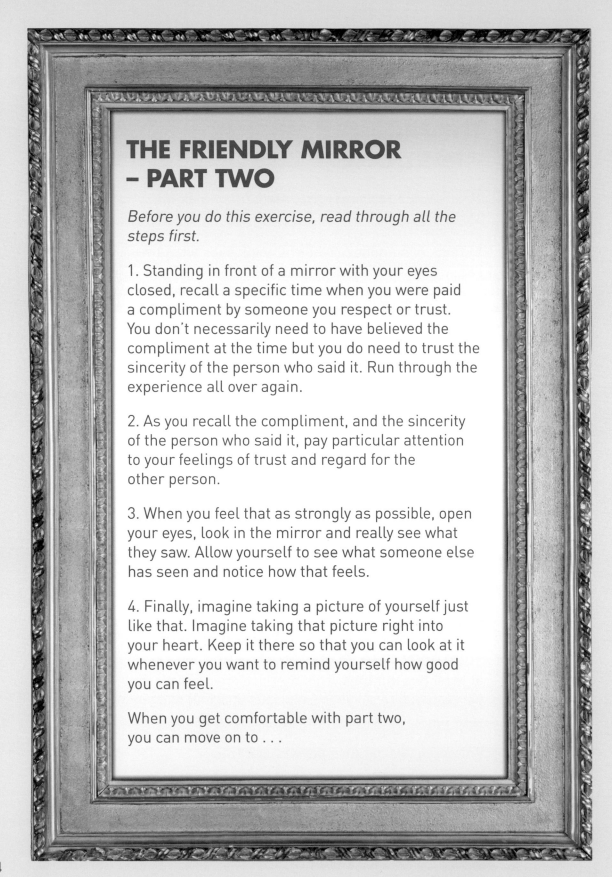

THE FRIENDLY MIRROR
– PART TWO

Before you do this exercise, read through all the steps first.

1. Standing in front of a mirror with your eyes closed, recall a specific time when you were paid a compliment by someone you respect or trust. You don't necessarily need to have believed the compliment at the time but you do need to trust the sincerity of the person who said it. Run through the experience all over again.

2. As you recall the compliment, and the sincerity of the person who said it, pay particular attention to your feelings of trust and regard for the other person.

3. When you feel that as strongly as possible, open your eyes, look in the mirror and really see what they saw. Allow yourself to see what someone else has seen and notice how that feels.

4. Finally, imagine taking a picture of yourself just like that. Imagine taking that picture right into your heart. Keep it there so that you can look at it whenever you want to remind yourself how good you can feel.

When you get comfortable with part two, you can move on to . . .

THE FRIENDLY MIRROR– PART THREE

Before you do this exercise, read through all the steps first.

1. Each day, spend at least one minute looking at your body in the mirror. In an ideal world, you will do this without clothes, but if that doesn't feel right at first, you may wear anything that reveals your basic shape.

2. Notice what thoughts come up, from 'This is stupid' to 'God, I hate my thighs' to 'Hmmm . . . not bad – not bad at all!'

3. Send love, approval and positive energy to the person in the mirror. Let them know that you're on their side, and that your love for them is not dependent on the size of their thighs.

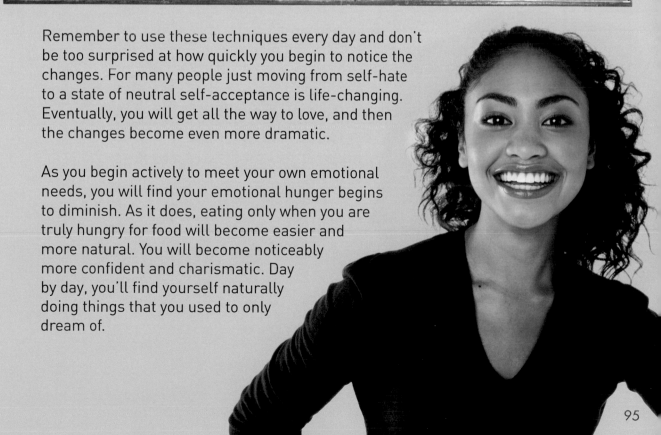

Remember to use these techniques every day and don't be too surprised at how quickly you begin to notice the changes. For many people just moving from self-hate to a state of neutral self-acceptance is life-changing. Eventually, you will get all the way to love, and then the changes become even more dramatic.

As you begin actively to meet your own emotional needs, you will find your emotional hunger begins to diminish. As it does, eating only when you are truly hungry for food will become easier and more natural. You will become noticeably more confident and charismatic. Day by day, you'll find yourself naturally doing things that you used to only dream of.

FREQUENTLY ASKED QUESTIONS
ABOUT 'OVERCOMING EMOTIONAL EATING'

Q. I'm hungry all the time, and I've been told it's just something I'd have to get used to. Could it also be partly emotional?

I would go so far as to say it's completely emotional. Being overweight is nearly always a symptom, and inescapable stress is nearly always the cause.

Yet book after book and programme after programme attempt to address the issue by telling you what you should or shouldn't eat. That's like trying to fix a broken leg by telling the person they shouldn't have fallen down. Instead of going outside yourself and asking the so-called diet experts, 'What should I eat?', you need to go inside and ask yourself 'What's eating me?'

The next time you're feeling overwhelmed, sad, angry, lonely or scared, put on the CD or use the exercises in this chapter to create a sense of instant calm and give yourself some unconditional love and approval. If you still want to eat after that, it's probably because you're actually hungry!

Q. I feel like I'm making real progress with this, but from time to time I feel overcome by a real need to eat an entire packet of biscuits. What do I do when I want to binge?

As some of your old patterns of overeating dissipate, it is not unusual for the odd craving to arise. When it does, you can proceed directly to Chapter Six and use the techniques to eliminate the cravings immediately!

CHRIS WILDE

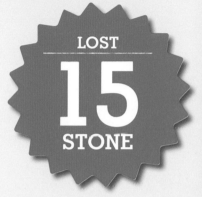

LOST
15
STONE

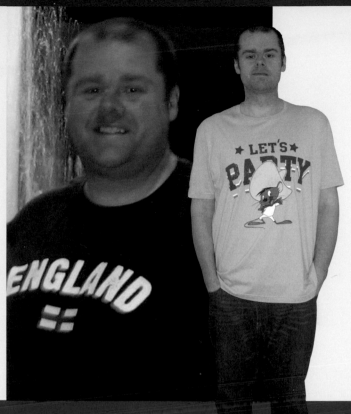

CHRIS'S STORY

I knew things were bad when I realized that I was just waiting to die. I had lost both my parents to cancer, I was struggling to find a good job after eighteen years in one I hated, and I was facing financial ruin. I barely had the energy to fight any more. Just when I was giving up, I discovered Paul's McKenna's weight-loss system.

I didn't know it at the time, but that discovery saved my life. I'd done plenty of diets in the past, and I'd lost large amounts of weight, but it always came back – plus a lot more. After twenty-five years of struggling with my weight, with this system it was suddenly easy to lose weight and keep it off. I was 386 pounds (27 and a half stone) when I started – I now weigh 175 pounds (12 and a half stone). I lost that weight in 14 months.

When I look back, I can hardly believe how much things have changed. Not only did the system help me to lose all that weight, but it helped me to build up my confidence. I've sorted out my financial difficulties and I found myself a great career – instead of driving buses and trucks, I assess the qualifications of drivers. I'm much happier in my work and I've kept the weight off!

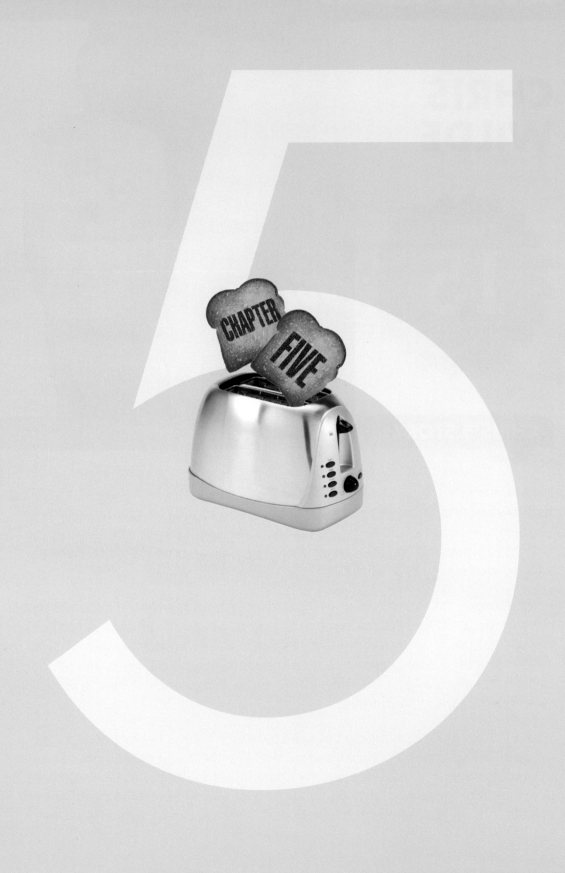

MAKE EXERCISE EASY AND SUPERCHARGE YOUR METABOLISM

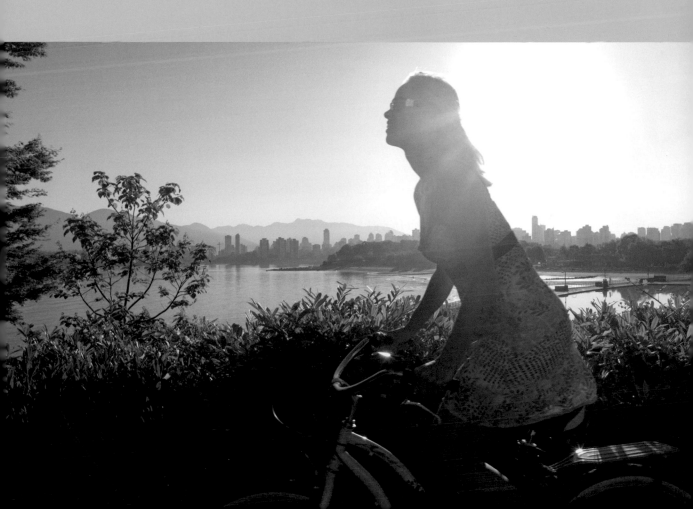

EXPLODING THE MYTH OF METABOLISM

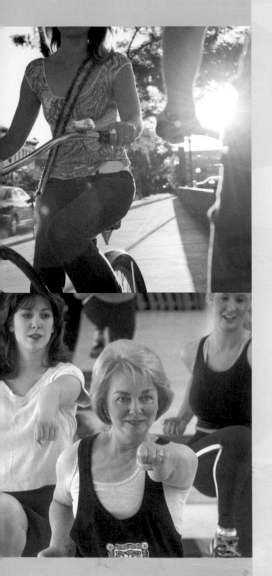

Have you ever heard someone say they can't lose weight because they have a 'slow' metabolism?

Your metabolism is the speed at which your body produces energy. The faster your metabolism, the faster your body does everything, from adjusting your body temperature to growing your fingernails. And more importantly for our purposes, the faster it will burn off any excess fat, regardless of whether that fat comes from a hearty roast beef platter or your hips, thighs and stomach.

The rate at which your metabolism is currently running is called your basal metabolic rate, and it is the primary determinant in how many calories your body will burn off throughout the day.

One of the great myths of the weight-loss world is the myth of metabolism, which says: *Certain people will find it more difficult to lose weight than others because of their genetically predetermined basal metabolic rate.*

However, the latest scientific research shows that your metabolic rate is not fixed – it can and will change throughout your life in response to how you eat and use your body.

Dr Susan Jebb is one of Britain's leading experts in the study of obesity. When discussing metabolism on one of my TV shows, she explained it like this:

When people go on a diet, their metabolism does change. Your body recognizes it's not getting as much food, as much fuel as it needs. The reduction in metabolic rate you see when people are dieting is essentially a very sensible evolutionary response to times of famine. If food was scarce, it made good sense to conserve energy, and so your metabolic rate decreases.

In other words, someone may really have a slow metabolism – but the reason it's so slow is because they've slowed it through endless dieting. In its effort to conserve energy when you're dieting, your body will slow all your energy systems down to a minimum. You'll feel sluggish and completely uninterested in exercise or any other physical activity.

To make matters worse, whatever lean muscle mass you do have will be consumed as your body literally eats itself to generate the extra energy it needs to function. So even if you are temporarily losing weight on the scale, you're not losing the right kind of weight – you're losing muscle.

Why is losing muscle bad? Because that lean muscle controls your basal metabolic rate – the number of calories your body can burn up for you while you're sitting in the office or home in bed.

There are very few 'sure things' in life, but I want to offer you one here:

If you continue to diet, you will gain weight and keep it on for life.

On the flip side, when you eat whenever you are hungry, your body learns it has plenty of fuel. It cranks up your metabolism so that energy can be used quickly and efficiently. Because it knows the energy will be replenished as needed, it doesn't bother to store any additional fat reserves, and you not only look thin but are filled with energy as well.

In the rest of this chapter, I will show you not only how to speed up your metabolism but how to 'supercharge' it too, enabling you to burn more fat and calories throughout the day and even while you sleep!

I USED PAUL'S TECHNIQUES TO HELP ME RUN A FIVE-KILOMETRE RACE. THE WEIGHT CAME OFF WITH HARDLY ANY EFFORT

KATHY TREVELYAN, TOUR GUIDE

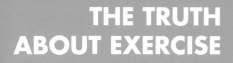

THE TRUTH ABOUT EXERCISE

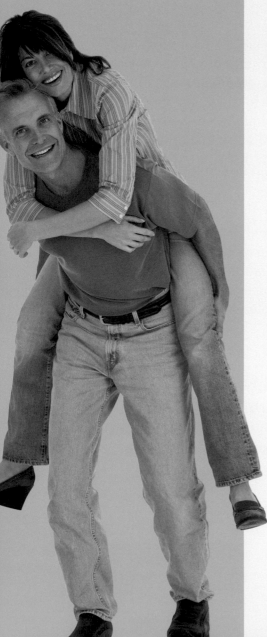

When I asked Dr Jebb if there was a 'secret' to supercharging your metabolism, she told me:

All you have to do is stop starving yourself and move your body more and your metabolism will increase. And the very best way to boost your metabolism is to become more active. Simply sitting in a chair uses up more energy than lying down. Standing up uses more energy than sitting down. Walking or climbing stairs all increase your metabolism and your energy needs. You can almost double your basic metabolic rate by being very physically active and burning off a lot of extra energy.

In other words, regular exercise will nearly double the speed of your metabolism. But before you throw your hands up in horror, realize that 'exercise' is simply this:

Anything you do that causes you to breathe more deeply than you normally would and/ or causes your heart rate to speed up.

Can you think of any enjoyable ways to get your heart pumping and to breathe more deeply than you are breathing now?

If so, you are already on your way to making exercise an easy and enjoyable part of your life.

When I ask people about exercise they think about running on a track or pumping iron. It always makes me laugh when people on my weight-loss seminars tell me they never exercise. 'Don't you get out of bed in the morning?' I ask them. 'How about walking around your home? Do you ever leave your flat or house? Does somebody carry you or do you do it on your own two feet?'

The fact is, you already 'exercise' all day every day, simply by moving your body. The key to supercharging your metabolism (and in so doing, increasing the rate at which your body burns up calories and fat) is simply to move more than you are currently doing. While the biggest exercise myth in the world is the idea of 'no pain no gain', the reality of exercise is this: **no effort, no gain; a little bit of effort, tremendous gain.**

Now let's take a look at some of the additional benefits of exercise. Studies have shown that regular exercisers not only lose weight, but they feel great. This is because exercise releases one of the best stress-reducing drugs available – your own natural endorphins. Here's how it works . . .

Your body does not distinguish between an emotional threat and a physical one. So even when you're just worrying about bad things happening, your body prepares to protect itself by fighting or running away – but often there is no one to fight and nowhere to run to. The body gets worked up but cannot find a way to release its tension.

Each time you exercise, you are helping your body release the tension of the stress response, making it feel calmer, safer and healthier. In addition, regular exercise triggers the body's natural impulse to rest, relaxation and recuperation, also known as the parasympathetic response. The parasympathetic response is the sweet, soft feeling you get in your muscles when you have finished some heavy work or vigorous movement.

You also feel a natural high caused by the release of endorphins, the body's natural opiates. That in turn positively affects your mood, making you emotionally clearer and more able to function well – to concentrate, to relax and to sleep soundly.

So any time you're feeling less than your best, you can give yourself an easy, positive boost by simply taking ten to fifteen minutes of brisk exercise – any movement (including walking) that speeds up your heart rate and gets you breathing more deeply than you are breathing right now.

HOW TO FAIL

Taking exercise helps you to build muscle, lose fat and feel great. It contributes to clearer skin, enhanced mental clarity, better athletic performance and an increased sex drive. Certain hormones released during exercise have been shown to slow and even reverse the ageing process.

So why aren't you already doing more of it?

Well, it's probably because in the past you thought about exercise and imagined yourself huffing and puffing on an exercise machine, listening to a maniacal aerobics instructor shouting 'feel the burn', or looking into a wall-sized mirror surrounded by people who look so much better than you that you just want to go home and throw up.

Or maybe you bought an exercise machine for yourself off the telly and you began to feel better the moment you ordered it. A few days later it arrived and you eagerly unpacked it, sure that the body of the model from the advert would be yours in just a few weeks' time. But within a month or so, your New Year's or birthday resolution became the world's most expensive clothes rack. In fact, most people put more and more clothes onto their exercise machines until they're so completely hidden that they don't have to look at them any more and remind themselves of what they're not doing.

In both cases the problem is that you have not yet linked pleasure to the thought of exercise.

It really is that simple – if you want to exercise regularly, you need to enjoy your moving of your body, both as you're doing it and after. Until you deliberately root out your negative associations with exercise and install new positive ones, you will continue to tell yourself you 'should' do it and beat yourself up for not listening.

As I guide you through this next exercise, we are going to make the idea of moving your body much more appealing, using the psychological power of vivid visualization and simple association to create a super-state of motivation to take exercise, which you can trigger whenever you want.

You are going to do this by creating an anchor, which will put you in touch with feeling great whenever you want. Since you already created a 'calm' anchor using the thumb and middle finger of your right hand, you may want to put this one on your left, or even use a different finger if you like. It's easy and inconspicuous and you can do it anywhere . . .

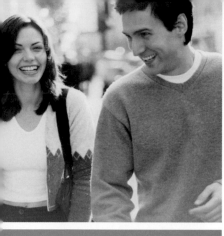
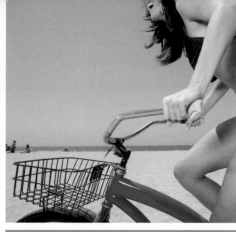
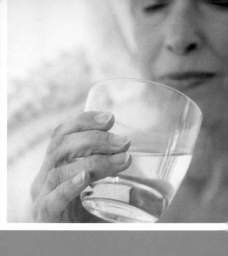
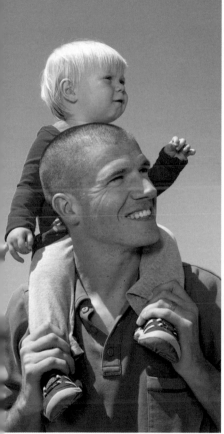

BUILD MUSCLE, LOSE FAT AND FEEL GREAT.

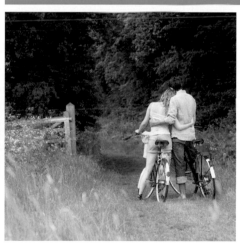
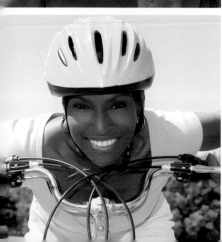
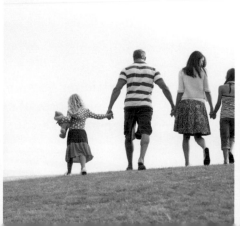
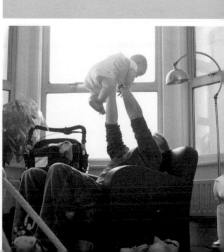

MOTIVATION POWER – PART ONE

In a moment we are going to remember some times when you felt totally motivated, or anything else that you REALLY enjoy doing. Then we are going to create an association between those feelings and this squeeze of your fingers by repeating them together, over and over again.

Before you do this exercise, read through all the steps first.

1 Rate on a scale of 1 to 10 how strong your motivation to exercise is. 1 is the weakest, 10 the strongest.

2 Think of something you are already motivated to do. It may be something you feel particularly passionate about, such as your favourite hobby or pastime, a political cause, being with a loved one or spending time with your family. If nothing springs to mind immediately, ask yourself, if you had won a lottery jackpot – how motivated would you be to go and collect the cheque? Or how motivated would you be to save the life of your closest friend? Or if the most attractive person in the world asked you out on a date – how motivated would you be to say yes?

3 Whatever motivates you most right now, I'd like you to visualize the scene – seeing it through your own eyes as though it's here now. See again what you would see, hear what you would hear and feel exactly how being motivated feels. Now notice all the details of the scene. Make the colours richer, bolder and brighter. Make the sounds clearer and the feelings stronger. As the feelings build to a peak, squeeze together your finger and thumb.

4 Keep going through that motivational movie. As soon as it finishes, start it again, all the time feeling that motivation and squeezing your thumb and finger together. See what you saw, hear what you heard, and feel that motivation.

5 STOP! Relax your fingers. Move about a bit.

Are you ready to test your motivation trigger? Squeeze your thumb and finger together and relive that good feeling now. It's important to realize it may not feel as intense, but you can increase your feelings of motivation every time you do this exercise.

MOTIVATION POWER – PART TWO

Before you do this exercise, read through all the steps first.

1 It's time to make the association between feeling motivated and moving your body. Squeeze your thumb and finger together and remember what it's like to feel motivated. Now imagine yourself moving your body easily and effortlessly throughout the day. Imagine things going perfectly, going exactly the way you want them to go, finding more and more opportunities to enjoy moving your body in enjoyable ways. See what you'll see, hear what you'll hear and feel how good it feels. As soon as you have done that, go through it again, still squeezing together your finger and thumb, permanently associating motivation to exercise.

2 Finally, on a scale of 1 to 10, how motivated do you feel to move your body? The higher the number, the easier you will find it to incorporate exercise into your daily routine. The lower the number, the more you need to practise the preceding technique. You can also listen to the mind-programming CD that comes with this book as often as you like. The more you listen, the more motivated to exercise you will become.

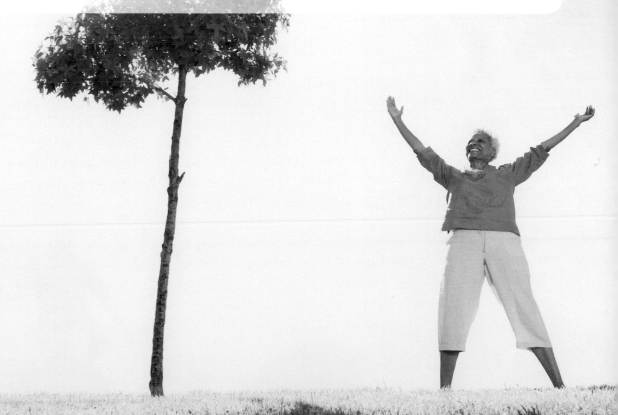

SIMPLE STEPS TO SUCCESS

Our bodies are made with muscles that are designed to be used. Because lots of us work at desks and travel by car, bus and train, we don't use our muscles as much as our ancestors used theirs. We have inherited all the healthy genes for fitness and a fast-burning metabolism, but we've fallen out of the habit of using them as much or as often as we could.

In an interesting study, researcher and author Dr James Hill discovered that the average number of steps taken per day by women between the ages of eighteen and fifty was only a little over 5,000. (For men, the average was closer to 6,000 steps a day.) Even more intriguingly, the study revealed that people who were overweight took 1,500 to 2,000 fewer steps a day than those who maintained a healthy weight.

Think about that for a moment – **only 2,000 extra steps a day can make the difference between being overweight and being slim!** That's about the distance it would take for you to walk four city blocks. The more steps you take, the more calories you use up, and the increased speed of your metabolism from those extra steps will continue to burn away your fat while you rest or sleep.

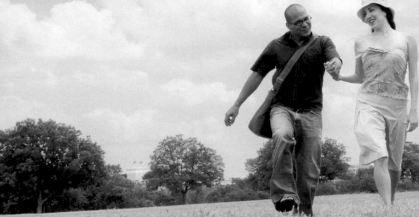

While some doctors recommend you maintain at least 10,000 steps a day, I have known people to make remarkable strides with their weight loss by increasing their step count to as much as 20,000 a day.

If you'd like to figure out how many steps you already walk each day, you can buy a simple pedometer (step counter) at almost any sports shop for about one pound. Just attach it to your clothing when you get started in the morning and find out how many steps you currently take in a typical day. Aim to increase the number of steps by 2,000 a week until you hit a comfortably maintainable target.

It's important to remember that no matter how much you want to change, it will still only happen one day at a time. You don't need to start a formal exercise programme (unless you want to clear up your skin, be less moody and have better sex), but you do need to move your body. Do it whenever you get the chance. Take the stairs instead of the lift. Park further away from the office and walk 2,000 extra steps to work. Move. Dance. Play sports. Have fun. You only have one body, so you might as well enjoy it!

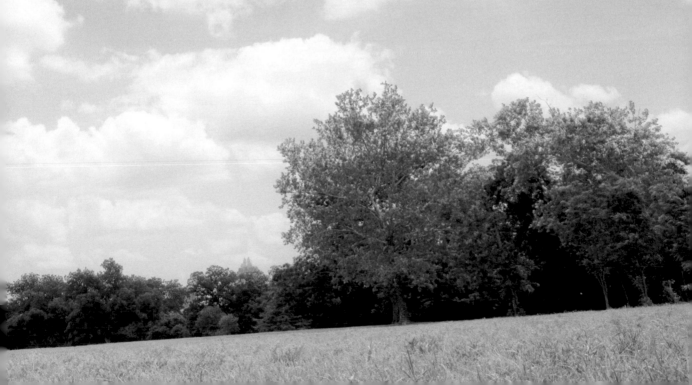

FREQUENTLY ASKED QUESTIONS ABOUT 'MAKE EXERCISE EASY AND SUPERCHARGE YOUR METABOLISM'

Q. Can I lose weight without any exercise?

Absolutely. As long as you are eating when you're hungry, eating what you actually want, enjoying each mouthful and stopping when you're full, you will lose weight.

But remember, it's virtually impossible not to exercise unless you're completely bedridden. (And even then you're probably breathing . . .) So given how easy it is to accelerate your weight loss by moving just a little bit more than you already do, why would you want to lose weight the slower way?

Q. How long will it take me to speed up my metabolism?

Your metabolism will begin to speed up the minute you start following the four golden rules. By gently introducing exercise into your routine, it will speed up even more. But be easy on yourself! I have noticed that when some people reach the desperation point, where they decide they have to lose weight immediately, they begin starving themselves, power walking and going to the gym all on the same day. When these people don't lose weight immediately (because they are driving their body into survival mode), they decide that it's all too much and they give up on the whole project.

Any task can be achieved if it's broken down into small enough chunks. That's why it's a good idea to choose a type and amount of exercise that you can succeed at easily and then increase it bit by bit each week. That way, you get to feel in control every step of the way.

Once you've succeeded the first three times, you'll continue doing it for life!

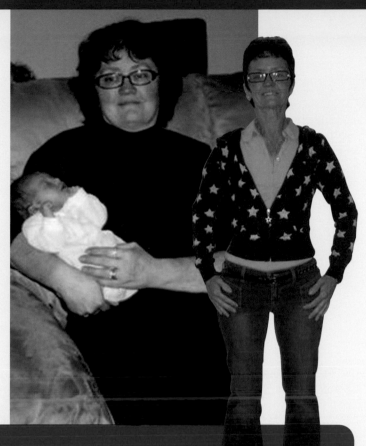

SHELLY FONTAINE

LOST
4 ½
STONE

SHELLY'S STORY

I started Paul's system in March 2008. I was 50 years old and 13 stone. For 20 years I'd been trying all kinds of diets; nothing worked. So I was sceptical, but I decided to follow what Paul was saying and see what happened.

I was busy caring for children and grandchildren at the time, and I hardly even noticed I was eating the leftovers from the children's plates when I was clearing up. I did what Paul suggested, and ate with my eyes closed and listened to what my stomach was saying. You really do taste the food more that way. I was shocked at how much food was left on the plate when I felt full. It was surprising how well it worked. I don't like exercise but I'd watch TV in the evening and move my legs up and down or sideways. It didn't matter what I was doing as long as I was moving them. This didn't feel like exercising, but it was.

This program is not just about weight loss, it's about changing your life. I am now the happiest I have ever been, and because of this, the children are happy too. Every chance I get I tell people that Paul McKenna gave me back my life. Thanks is not enough!

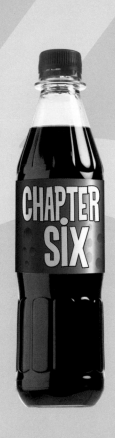

CRAVING BUSTERS

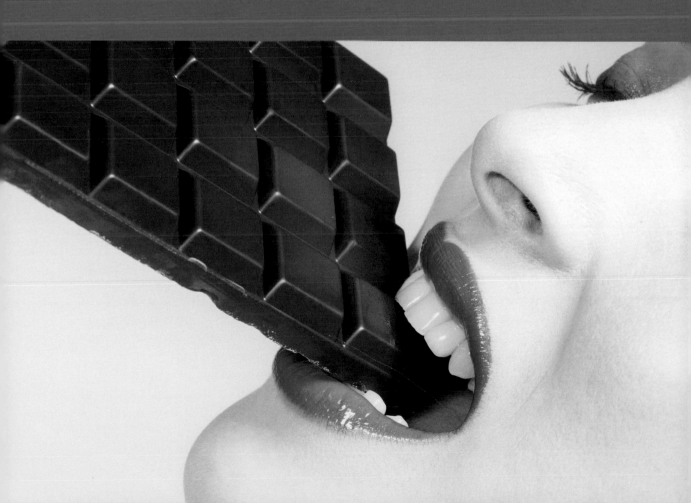

HOW TO TAKE CONTROL OF YOUR CRAVINGS

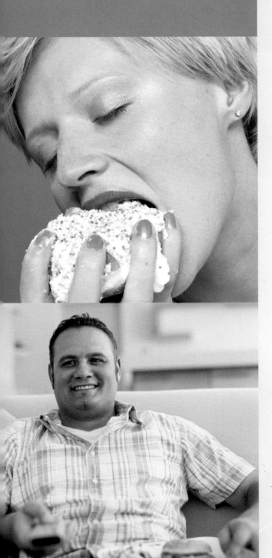

One of the main concerns people have about using my system is that I am going to somehow trick them into hating their favourite foods and they'll constantly feel like they are missing out. Nothing could be further from the truth – as you've already learned, in my system there are NO forbidden foods. As long as you're hungry and you fancy it, it's yours.

However, if you can't stop once you start or you can't resist a food even when you're not hungry, then in that moment you are out of control. If you have to demolish the whole bar of chocolate or scarf down the entire bag of chips, the food is in charge and not you. The techniques in this chapter will help put you back in charge of your body, your eating and your life.

Now, if you have ever had a craving, you know that it feels like it needs to be satisfied immediately. In addition, most cravings are for a specific food, like chocolate, pizza or cheesecake, as opposed to a more general hunger.

Here's all you need to know:

**Any craving you may have felt
is a learned behaviour.**

That means you weren't born with it, and if you learned it, you can unlearn it, often in a matter of minutes.

There are two techniques in this chapter. If you are in the midst of a food craving, I'm about to share with you a startlingly simple way you can reduce or even eliminate that craving in less than two minutes. If you would like to reprogram your mind to stop a particular craving for ever, you can skip ahead to the second technique . . .

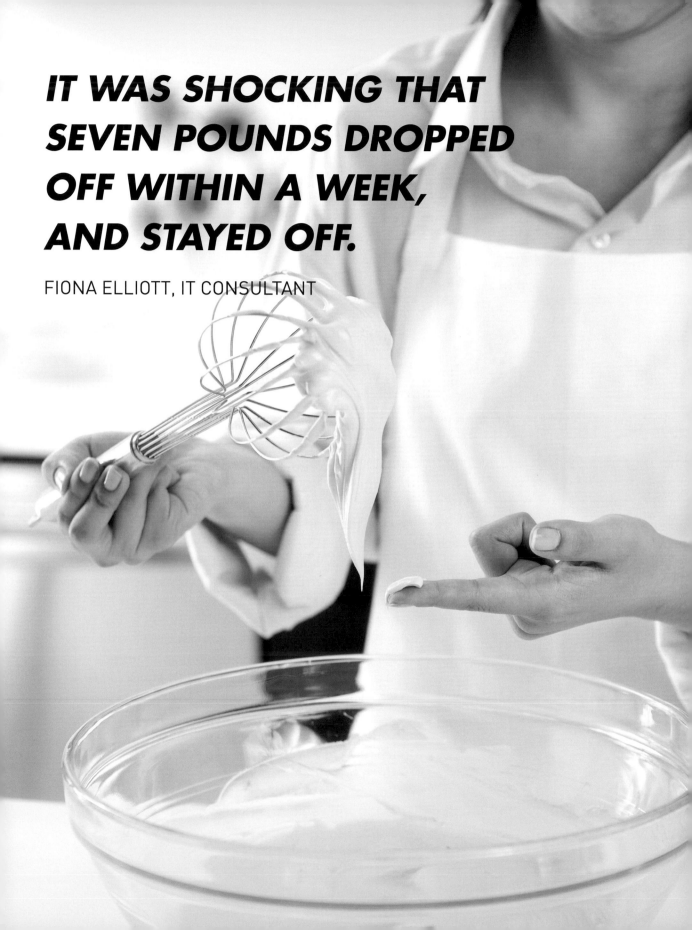

IT WAS SHOCKING THAT SEVEN POUNDS DROPPED OFF WITHIN A WEEK, AND STAYED OFF.

FIONA ELLIOTT, IT CONSULTANT

THE TAPPING TECHNIQUE

This amazing technique was developed by Dr Roger Callahan, author of **Tapping the Healer Within**.

In one of the television programmes I did on weight loss, we featured a lady named Lizzie who drank four litres of cola every single day. We asked her to take part in a dramatic experiment – to go 'cold turkey' and stop drinking cola completely. The results were distressing. Lizzie experienced constant cravings, and after only a few days she had become depressed and hysterical.

At that point I called her and guided her through the tapping technique I am about to share with you. Amazingly, within a few minutes the crying and the cravings had completely stopped. For the first time she could remember, Lizzie felt in control. When the cravings came back, as I had told her might happen, she was now able to switch them off at will.

The first day she had to tap them away almost a dozen times. By the next day it was down to eight, and by the end of the week the cravings were coming up only one or two times a day. At the time of writing, Lizzie has not drunk cola once since she learned the tapping sequence you are about to learn. Better still, she hasn't even experienced a craving for over two years.

If you are feeling a strong craving for a particular food right now and you want to reduce or even eliminate it immediately, just follow my instructions completely and your craving will vanish. This process may seem

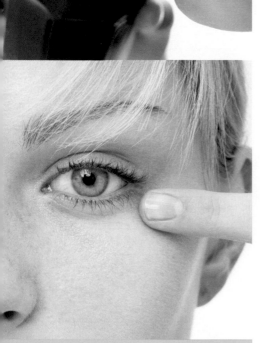

a bit strange at first, but it works. You will need to be able to really concentrate for a few minutes, as it is important that you continue thinking about the food you have chosen as you go through this process and reduce the craving.

What we are about to do involves tapping on certain acupuncture points on your body. The code for any craving is stored like a computer programme in your brain. By thinking about the food you are craving while tapping on each point in exactly the sequence I am about to describe, you reset your brain's operating software to bypass your cravings so you can easily get on with your life.

BYPASS YOUR CRAVINGS AND GET ON WITH YOUR LIFE.

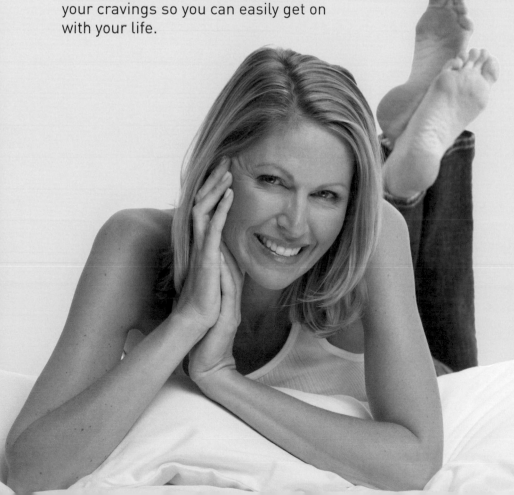

TAPPING INTO THE THIN WITHIN

Before you do this technique, read through each step so you know exactly what to do.

1 I want you get the biggest desire for your favourite craving food. Now, rate your craving on a scale of 1 to 10, with 1 being the lowest and 10 the highest. This is important, because in a moment we will find out how much you've reduced it.

2 Now take two fingers of either hand and tap about ten times under your collarbone while you continue to think about your craving.

3 Now tap under your eye ten times.

4 Now tap under your collarbone again.

5 Place your other hand in front of you and tap on the back of it between your ring finger and your little finger. Continue to think about your craving food as you do this and each of the steps which follow:

- Close your eyes and open them.
- Keep your head still, keep tapping and look down to the right, then down to the left.
- Keep tapping and rotate your eyes round 360 degrees clockwise, and now 360 degrees anti-clockwise.

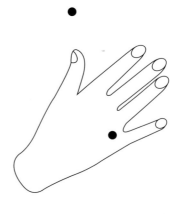

Remember to keep thinking about the food you were craving as you do this!

- Now hum the first few lines of 'Happy Birthday' out loud.
- Count out loud from 1 to 5.
- Once again hum the first few lines of 'Happy Birthday' out loud.

6 Stop and check – on a scale from 1 to 10, what number is your craving at now?

If it hasn't completely gone yet, just repeat this sequence again until it does. It may take as many as two or even three times before you have completely eliminated the craving, although most people report getting their craving down to a manageable level on their first or second try. You may even find that it is gone completely.

If it ever comes back, you can repeat this process as often as you like, or go through the Craving Buster Number Two to reprogram your craving away for ever.

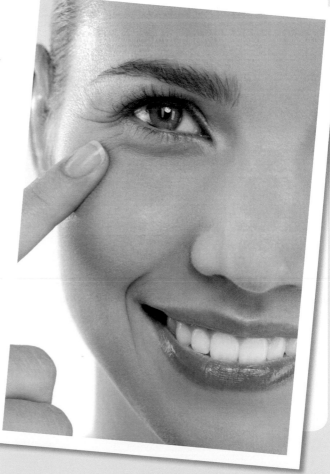

THE COMPULSION DESTROYER

Before you do this technique, read through each step so you know exactly what to do.

While the tapping technique you have just learned can be used to reduce and ultimately even eliminate cravings over time, this next technique can eliminate food compulsions for ever in just a few applications. In fact, I regularly demonstrate this technique on television and in my seminars to help someone who considers themselves to be a chocolate 'addict' to become unwilling to eat chocolate ever again – in less than two minutes!

I am now going to show you how to do the same thing for yourself – how you can stop yourself from ever wanting to eat a particular food again. Most people choose chocolate, bread, biscuits or some other food that has turned from an occasional treat to uplift your spirits to a heavy anchor round your hips and thighs.

Remember, only do this next technique if you genuinely want to stop eating a particular food for good! If you just want to reduce your craving, go back to 'Tapping into the thin within'. Read through this technique in its entirety before you do it.

1. Think of a food you hate – one that really disgusts you. (A woman on one of my trainings who swore that she loved to eat everything finally agreed that she found the idea of eating a plate of human hair repulsive.)

2. Next, I want you to vividly imagine there is a big plate of the food you hate in front of you. Now imagine smelling and then eating the food that you hate, as you squeeze the thumb and little finger of either hand together. Really imagine the texture of it on your mouth as you squeeze your thumb and little finger together. Imagine the taste of it, squeezing your thumb and little finger together until you feel utterly revolted. When you are feeling a bit nauseous, stop and relax your fingers.

3 Next, I want you to think of the food you are going to stop eating. When you think of it, notice that you can imagine what a plate of it looks like.

4 Now, make that picture of the food you like bigger, bigger and brighter. Make it huge, until it's bigger than you, and make it even bigger than that. Continue making it bigger and bigger and bring it closer and closer and then pass it through you and out the other side. (Most people say that it feels a bit weird to pass the picture through your body – like when a ghost passes through your body in the Harry Potter stories.)

5 Ready? Squeeze your thumb and finger together and remember the taste of the food you hate, while at the same time imagining eating some of the food you like. Now, imagine the food you like is mixed in with the food you hate. Imagine eating the two foods together, the food you love and the food you hate. Keep imagining the taste and texture of the two together. Keep eating them in your mind, a big plate, swallow them down, as you squeeze your thumb and little finger together. That's it, eat even more, more and more until you can't eat any more, then stop.

6 Think about the food you used to like and notice how it's different now.

You can repeat this process as often as you like until you have completely eliminated your desire for that particular food. You will no longer be a slave to your cravings.

FREQUENTLY ASKED QUESTIONS ABOUT 'CRAVING BUSTERS'

Q. What if I drink a lot? Can I still lose weight?

Let's get really honest here – you're not fat because of what you drink. After all, there are plenty of thin alcoholics. The real issue with excessive drinking isn't weight gain, it's unconsciousness – and I'm not talking about drinking until you pass out!

Most people drink so they don't have to deal with what's really going on in their lives – but now that you've begun this system, what's really going on in your life is a process of continual, positive change. I would suggest that, at least at first, don't drink when you eat and don't eat when you are drinking, but if you do, just make sure to continue to follow the four golden rules.

(If you think you've got a drinking problem, then seek help from an appropriate professional.)

Q. I was doing really well but then I had a binge over the weekend – is it worth carrying on or should I wait until I've got my life more under control?

Your life will never be under control until you begin to control yourself – and every one of the tools in this system will help you. Following the four golden rules, learning to manage your emotions and moving your body are all disciplines – but they get easier and easier the more you do them.

In addition, the more control you gain over your eating, the more positive benefits you'll begin to experience in other areas of your life. It's not uncommon for people to report less stress, greater happiness and even increased income as a result of applying this system over time.

As for the binge, forgive yourself and move on. It's not unusual and it's not your fault. As some of the old patterns of overeating dissipate, cravings arise. But now that you have the tools from this chapter, you'll be able to tap, tap, tap them away!

MONIQUE SMITH

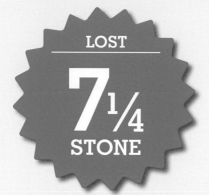

LOST

7 ¼

STONE

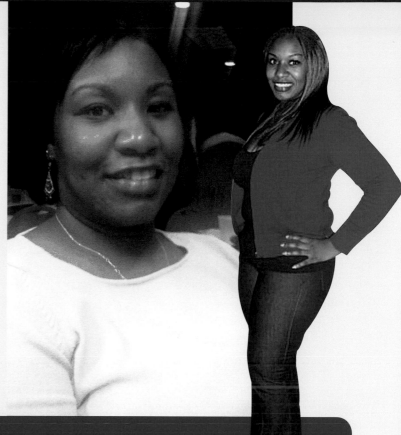

MONIQUE'S STORY

I'm so happy to share my success story with everyone. I started using the I Can Make You Thin technique in June 2008. It really made so much sense to me just to give it a shot, and so I did – and it changed my life. I have lost a total of 104 pounds and I look and feel better than I have over the last seven years. Now that I have portion control and have lost the weight, I have the energy to exercise, which has helped me tone up my body. I am extremely happy. I have some more pounds to lose but I am still very happy with where I am now.

I started a Facebook weight-loss challenge about a month ago and I have about 1,000 members on there now. I want to be a weight-loss icon and an inspiration to others. I have made it my mission to help as many people as I can to get back on track to healthy eating and to get that extra weight off them!

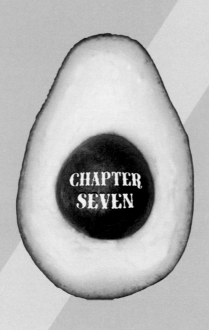

CHAPTER
SEVEN

THE FINAL PIECE OF THE WEIGHT-LOSS PUZZLE

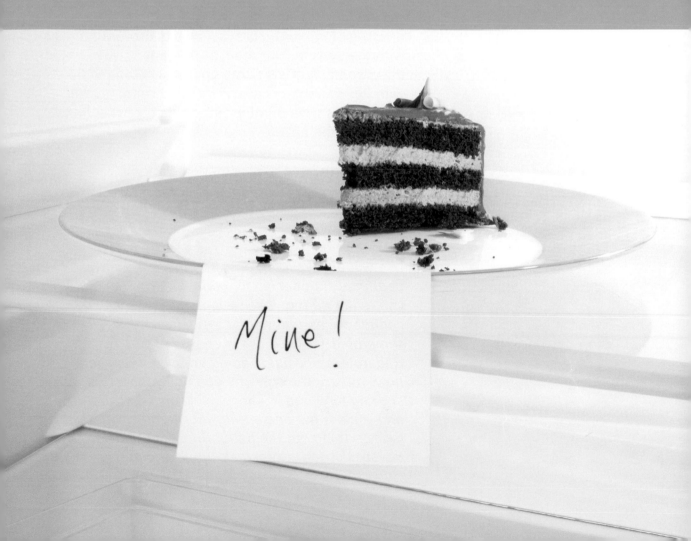

STOPPING SELF-SABOTAGE BEFORE IT STARTS

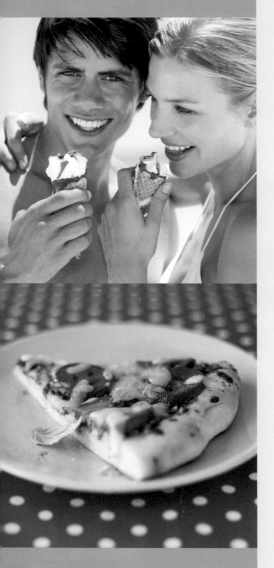

Remember, if you want to lose weight and keep it off for life, all you need to do is:

1. Eat when you're hungry.

2. Eat what you want, not what you think you should eat.

3. Enjoy every mouthful.

4. Stop when you think you're full.

So what could possibly stop you from following these four simple principles?

I worked with a woman on one of our one-day weight-loss events I'll call Sheila. She had read the book, listened to the CD and actually lost nearly a stone in the first six weeks of working with the system. But then, as she put it, 'life intervened'. A crisis came up in her relationship with her daughter, her car stopped running and she had a series of minor illnesses over the course of the next few months.

'The system,' she said, 'stopped working.'

While I felt sympathy for her, I knew that what she really needed to hear was this:

Life will always intervene, and there will always be things clamouring for your attention. But if you really want to lose weight, increase your confidence and feel great inside, you have to remember that you are in charge of you. Regardless of what is going on in your life right now, you are the only one opening your mouth and shoving food into it when you're not really hungry, and you are the one letting your mind pay attention to everything but the delightful sensations and flavours of your breakfast, lunch and dinner.

The system never stops working – you stop following it.

And the good news is, you can restart your weight loss right now by simply tuning in to your body, noticing where you are on the hunger scale, and following the four golden rules day by day.

To my delight, Sheila came back on another course six months later, three stone lighter but, far more importantly, glowing from the inside out with a sense of achievement and new possibility.

When I talked to the 29 per cent of people who couldn't get the system to work for them, it always came down to the same thing – they weren't following the system.

Sometimes, it was an active distrust:

- 'I thought you were going to make me stop eating cream cakes and I love them.'

- 'He can't really mean eat whenever you're hungry – I'll just use the system during my one meal a day.'

- 'I'm sure he didn't mean eat what you actually want all the time – surely he just wants us to treat ourselves from time to time. I'll stick with the baked skinless chicken breasts but I'll have a bit of whipped cream on my low-fat no-sugar-added diet cardboard cake.'

- 'Dieting's not that bad – after all, lost weight before my wedding by starving myself. I'll just use this as a set of guidelines for making my diet work better.'

If any of this sounds like you, the choice is simple: follow my system completely and lose weight easily, or throw this book on the pile with the other failed diet manuals. I don't know any psychological system or drug that works for everyone all the time, but I can absolutely guarantee you that it won't work if you don't follow it.

But what was really interesting to me were the people who didn't even realize they weren't following the system. Consciously, they were completely engaged and committed, but unconsciously they were carrying hidden beliefs that were sabotaging their success.

Many people who hear this idea immediately recognize that it's true for them, but don't know what to do about it. Others ask: 'But if my self-sabotage beliefs are unconscious, how can I know what they are?'

The good news is: you don't need to know what your unconscious beliefs are in order to change them.

CREATING WHOLENESS

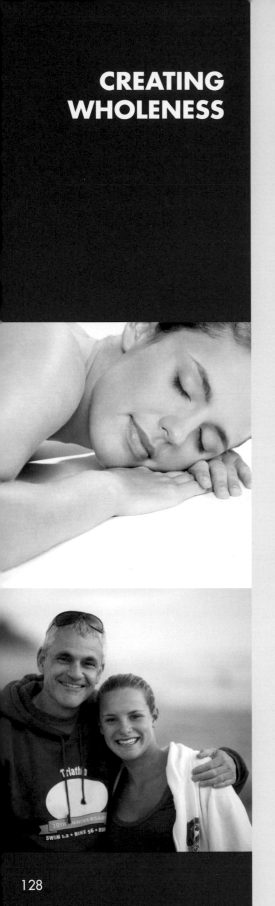

Have you ever heard people talk about 'a part' of themselves? For example, they might say, 'A part of me wants to go to the cinema, but part of me wants to stay at home,' or, 'Part of me wants to get my work done, but part of me wants to skive off for the day.'

It's not as though there actually are 'parts' inside you. It's simply different aspects of your consciousness that are temporarily in conflict. And when two or more 'parts' of you are butting heads, the one that's strongest at that time will determine your behaviour and the eventual outcome.

Sometimes you will hear it as: 'I want to ask that person out, but I am afraid I'll get rejected' or 'I feel torn – I know what I need to do but I can't bring myself to do it'. So one part of them wants to take action or to be in a relationship, and another part is trying to protect against the pain of rejection.

What about you? Is there a part of you that really wants to lose weight, but another part that's not so sure? Do you find yourself firmly resolving that this time, you're really going to do it, only to go unconscious and go back to trying to satisfy your emotional hunger with chip butties?

When this happens, it's a bit like driving down the street with one foot on the accelerator and the other on the brake – you may make progress, but you won't enjoy the journey and neither will anyone around you.

Over the years I have heard a vast array of reasons for self-sabotage of my system, and even though they might not be logical, they serve an important purpose for the person who thinks them:

- 'I have failed so many times in the past, I am worried that I will lose weight, but then put it all back on and feel really disappointed'.

- 'I had an affair because I was attractive and nearly lost my marriage. I am worried that if I lose weight it will happen again.'

- 'This is so simple it's too good to be true. I have spent years trying to lose weight and it's been very difficult. I will be furious with myself if this works, for all the time and effort I have wasted.'

- 'I was abused and it was because I was beautiful and thin. I am frightened to lose weight in case it happens again.'

Even though these may not sound very logical reasons to stay overweight, they make perfect sense to anyone who understands how the unconscious works. Your unconscious mind is not logical, it's purposeful – and its primary purpose is to ensure your survival and safety, no matter what the price.

This is the most important thing for you to know:

Every part of you has a positive intention.

The part that wants to lose weight wants you to feel good about yourself and be healthy. The part that's worried you'll fail and feel disappointed is

trying to protect you from feelings of unhappiness. Even though they are taking you in seemingly opposite directions, they both share the same overriding intention: they both want the best for you. And when you apply the technique I am about to share with you, they will begin to work together for your highest good.

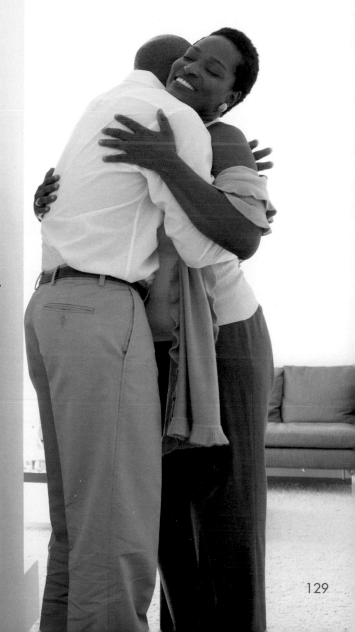

129

CREATING INTEGRATED SELF-BELIEF

1 Identify the two conflicting beliefs or positions within your mind. For example, part of you might want to lose weight, but another part of you might want to stay overweight because it believes that will keep you safe. Or maybe you are scared you will fail and feel upset, so you might as well sabotage your attempts now and get it over with.

2 Place your hands out in front of you, palms up. Imagine the part that wants to lose weight in your right hand and the 'sabotage' part in your left.

3 Ask each part in turn what its positive intention is for you, in wanting what it wants. Continue asking until you clearly recognize that at some level they both want the same thing. Even if it feels like you are just making it up, going through this process will create dramatic changes in your levels of confidence and self-belief.

Example:

WEIGHT LOSS => MORE ATTRACTIVE => BETTER HEALTH => SUCCESS!

SABOTAGE => MORE CAUTIOUS => FEEL SAFE => SUCCESS!

4 Imagine a new, 'super part' in between your hands with the combined resources of both your weight loss and your sabotage. So, for example, can you lose weight in a way that makes you feel safe?

5 Moving only as quickly as you can, bring your hands together until the two separate parts become one with the super part.

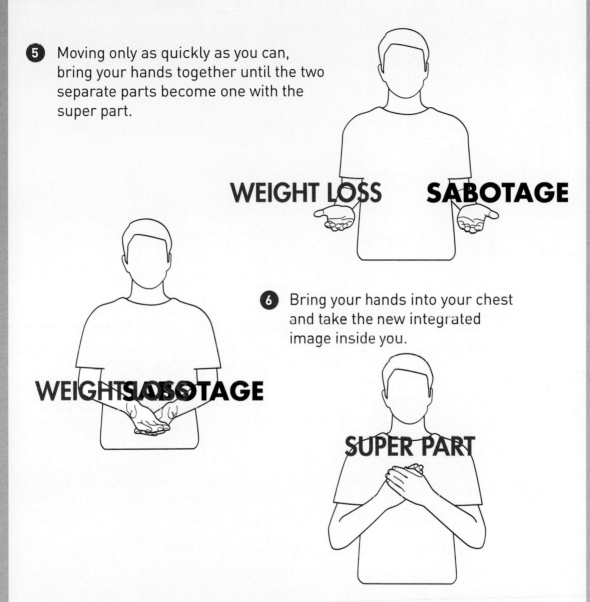

WEIGHT LOSS   SABOTAGE

WEIGHT LOSS SABOTAGE

6 Bring your hands into your chest and take the new integrated image inside you.

SUPER PART

As you practise this technique, you will find it becomes easier and easier to resolve every internal conflict in this way. And when all parts of yourself are aligned and moving in the same direction, you will have become focused like a laser beam on whatever you decide to do!

This technique is used with the permission of Dr Richard Bandler.

FREQUENTLY ASKED QUESTIONS ABOUT 'THE FINAL PIECE OF THE WEIGHT-LOSS PUZZLE'

Q. It's been nearly a week and I haven't lost any weight yet. What am I doing wrong?

Do you mean besides the fact that you're weighing yourself before the first two weeks are up?

There's an old story about a farmer who gave his daughter a packet of seeds to plant so that she would learn about the natural order of planting and nurturing what you most want to see develop and grow. Yet even though he had given her some of the simplest growing seeds available, nothing new ever seemed to emerge from the field.

One day, the farmer noticed his daughter digging up the seeds and holding them up to the light. When he asked her what she was doing, she told him she wanted to see if there was anything growing yet. What she didn't realize was that each time she dug up a seed, she was preventing it from evolving at its natural pace.

In the same way, if you keep weighing yourself without allowing time for these seeds to take root in your unconscious, the only things that will grow are your stomach, hips and thighs.

Q. What do I do if I fall off the wagon?

It's perfectly OK to make mistakes. As a baby did you walk on your first attempt? When you learned to ride a bike did you wobble at first and come off a few times? Have the world's greatest achievers made mistakes on their journeys to success?

I would assume that in the first few weeks it's highly likely you will have a slip and overeat, or temporarily forget to follow the rules. It's fine, just return to following the rules again. Some people use a little slip to beat themselves up and tell themselves that once again they have failed; they console themselves with a binge or just give up on the system, resigned to the fact that they will always be fat.

Not this time! Simply go back to following the rules, eat when you are hungry, enjoy each mouthful and when you suspect you are full, stop!

As for the binge, forgive yourself and move on. It's not unusual and it's not your fault. As some of the old patterns of overeating dissipate, cravings arise. But now that you have the tools from this chapter, you'll be able to tap, tap, tap them away!

Once you've succeeded the first three times, you'll continue doing it for life!

Q. I started losing weight, but now it's stopped. What do I do?

1. Are you eating whenever you're hungry?

2. Are you eating what you actually want, not what you think you should?

3. Are you eating consciously and enjoying every mouthful?

4. Are you stopping when you think you're full (even if there's still food on your plate)?

If you can honestly answer yes to each of these questions, then the secret is to slow your eating speed down even more!

Here's how it works: your stomach expands and contracts according to how much food you put into it. In the past, you were eating so fast you couldn't hear your body's full signal. Consequently, you overate and expanded your stomach, thereby creating a need for more food to make you full. When you began to slow down your eating speed, you became conscious of what you were eating as you were eating it, and were able to notice the full signal much quicker. You ate less food, your stomach contracted and you needed less and less food to become full.

However, our bodies are highly adaptive. By now, you may have become so used to eating at your new, slower speed that you have once again gone unconscious about what's going on with your body as you eat. By slowing down even more, you will once again 'trick yourself awake', and be able to tune in again to your body's satiation signals.

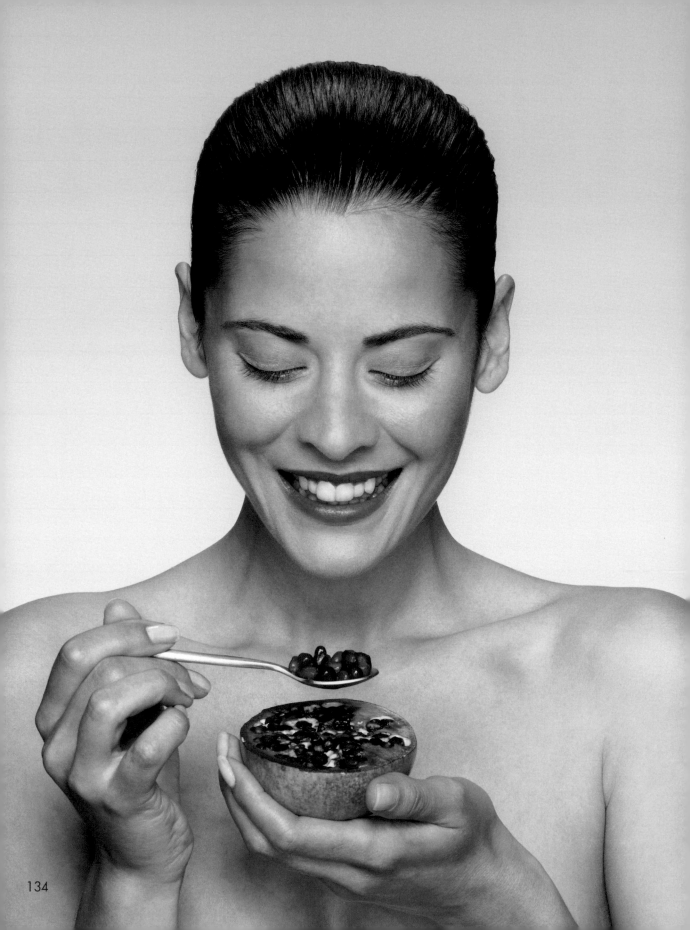

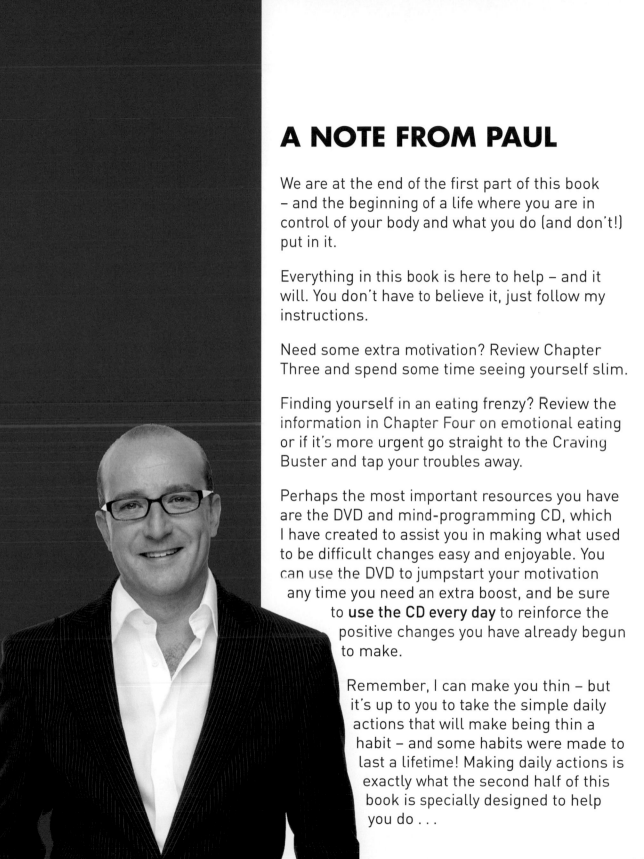

A NOTE FROM PAUL

We are at the end of the first part of this book – and the beginning of a life where you are in control of your body and what you do (and don't!) put in it.

Everything in this book is here to help – and it will. You don't have to believe it, just follow my instructions.

Need some extra motivation? Review Chapter Three and spend some time seeing yourself slim.

Finding yourself in an eating frenzy? Review the information in Chapter Four on emotional eating or if it's more urgent go straight to the Craving Buster and tap your troubles away.

Perhaps the most important resources you have are the DVD and mind-programming CD, which I have created to assist you in making what used to be difficult changes easy and enjoyable. You can use the DVD to jumpstart your motivation any time you need an extra boost, and be sure to **use the CD every day** to reinforce the positive changes you have already begun to make.

Remember, I can make you thin – but it's up to you to take the simple daily actions that will make being thin a habit – and some habits were made to last a lifetime! Making daily actions is exactly what the second half of this book is specially designed to help you do . . .

Love Food
Lose Weight

What follows here is your support tool. Having shared this system with over half a million people in a single year, I found that this was the one thing people kept asking for – a way of keeping track of progress and keeping on track when old patterns once again begin to rear their ugly heads. Based on your feedback, I created the 90-day Success Journal to provide extra support for those of you who want that little something extra. Now, for the first time, I Can Make You Thin and the 90-day Success Journal are available together in this single volume.

This is an amazing self-guiding journal that will take you step by step through a personal mind-body makeover that will help you transform you relationship with food and your body forever!

It's not just the act of writing things down or ticking boxes that focuses your thoughts and behaviours for success. It's the commitment you are making to yourself as you change your old routine and do something different that will disrupt the negative patterns and set you on a new course to a healthier way of eating and a happier way of life!

If you've never kept a journal before, prepare to be amazed at the difference it will make in your life.

To your success,

Paul McKenna

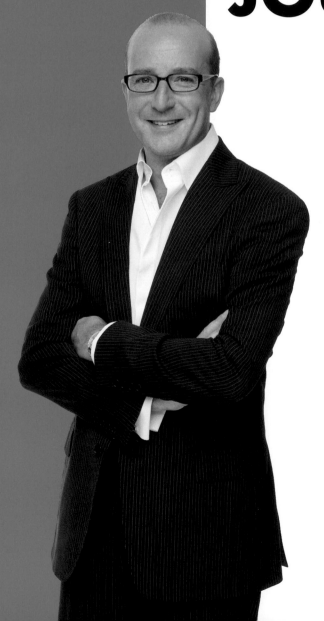

90-DAY SUCCESS JOURNAL

KEEPING A JOURNAL WILL ABSOLUTELY CHANGE YOUR LIFE IN WAYS YOU'VE NEVER IMAGINED.

OPRAH WINFREY

KEEPING A JOURNAL

The weight-loss system you are about to embark upon is the most successful in the world. If it were a pill I could sell it to a drug company for a billion dollars. But it's not a pill, it's a system – a system so simple that, at first, most people can't believe it will work for them.

The best thing is, you don't have to believe in it and there's no willpower required. All you have to do is just follow my instructions and your life will dramatically change for the better.

This is your support tool – a 90-day success journal, which will support and guide you over the next three months until you've firmly established the new habits of relating to food and your body that will last you for a lifetime.

A recent study by Dr Ben Fletcher showed that when people change their routines they naturally lose weight, even though they aren't told to diet or exercise. To help you change your routine, I have packed this journal with simple, fun activities that will interrupt your old patterns of thinking and behaviour and help you to create and maintain new ones.

Here's how it all works . . .

WEEKLY THEMES

Each week, you will be introduced to a theme, ranging from understanding emotional eating to lightening up and having more fun in your life. These weekly themes relate to the key sections in the earlier part of the book.

DAILY THOUGHTS AND ACTIVITIES

Each day, I will share with you one of my favourite quotes, along with a simple thought or exercise you can do to solidify the changes you are making in how you think and act around food. Then you will find an eight-item 'Success Checklist'. These activities are the keys to your success:

1 Eating when you are hungry

2 Eating what you **really** want

3 Eating consciously

4 Stopping when you are full

5 Drinking water

6 Moving your body

7 Listening to the mind-programming CD

8 Doing the Friendly Mirror exercise (see pages 92–5)

It is important for you to know that while following the first four golden rules is at the heart of my system, **it is not necessary for you to do every single thing on every single day in order to succeed**. In fact, I would be amazed if you did. This is about progress, not perfection – and as long as you are doing most things on most days, you will make tangible progress towards your goals.

TODAY AND TOMORROW

Underneath the success checklist, I've made space for you to make notes about one positive thing you've noticed today and at least one thing you're looking forward to tomorrow. Don't underestimate the power of these two simple observations. What you focus on in life expands, and by focusing on your positive experiences and positive expectancies, you will find yourself drawing more and more of what you want into your life.

'REVIEW AND RENEW' DAYS

Every seventh day is set aside for review and renewal. This will give you a chance to reflect back on the week just gone and look forward to the week ahead. There are five things to record on your review days:

1 The best things that happened

2 The most challenging things that happened

3 Any new behaviours

4 What you learned

5 Your top priorities for the week ahead

You can see a sample 'Review and renew' day filled in on page 140.

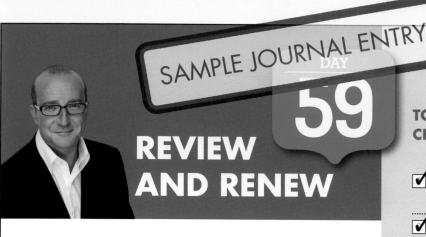

DAY 59

REVIEW AND RENEW

REFLECT UPON YOUR PRESENT BLESSINGS, OF WHICH EVERY MAN HAS MANY; NOT UPON YOUR PAST MISFORTUNES, OF WHICH ALL MEN HAVE SOME.

CHARLES DICKENS

Did you enjoy your week of eating mindfully? It doesn't have to end today – as you move into the final month of our time together, mindfulness can be a powerful ally as you continue to reprogram your mind and body to be naturally thin. Take some time today to ask and answer these questions . . .

1. The best things that happened this week were:

Followed the rules 5 of 6 days; great meeting at work on Tuesday

2. My biggest challenges this week were:

Binged on cake at party; the argument(!)

3. I did these things for the first time:

Took the dogs for a walk because I actually wanted some exercise

4. What I learned was:

One bad day doesn't have to ruin my week

5. My top three priorities for the week ahead are:

a. *Drink more water*

b. *Prepare sales reports for work*

c. *Spend more time doing the mirror exercise*

TODAY'S SUCCESS CHECKLIST

☑ I ate when I was hungry

☑ I ate what I really wanted

☑ I ate consciously

☑ I stopped when full
   Yaaay

☑ I drank water

[6] I moved my body

[7] I listened to the CD
   Load CD into iPod

☑ I did the mirror exercise

One **Positive Thing**
I Noticed Today . . .

I think this really is working – I didn't

even notice the doughnuts had been and

gone at work until the end of the day

What I'm **Looking Forward To**
Tomorrow . . .

Meeting Brian for drinks down the pub

CHECK-IN DAYS

Spread throughout the journal you will find six 'check-in' days. These are the only days I want you to weigh yourself. In fact, this is the one part of the journal you could skip altogether – looking great and feeling wonderful will always be a better measure of your progress than the numbers on a scale.

As I said in part one, you cannot get an accurate reading on your weight loss by checking every day. By taking a full two weeks between weigh-ins, you will get a sense of your real progress, instead of just tracking the daily weight fluctuations that everyone goes through regardless of how overweight or thin they already are.

On each check-in day, you will have another opportunity to read testimonials from people who have successfully used my system to lose weight and free up their bodies and minds from the patterns of obsessive dieting, emotional eating and faulty programming that kept them from living happily and at their desired weight.

The final testimonial in the book will be . . . yours!

YOUR OWN SUCCESS STORY

In order to prepare yourself to be truly amazed at how well you do on this system, I want you to take a picture of yourself as you look now and paste or tape it into the 'Before' box on day 90. Don't worry if you hate being photographed or think you look terrible. By the time you've finished, this will be your favourite picture in the world – a reminder of how things used to be and how far you've come in such a relatively short period of time.

If you've decided to weigh yourself on the check-in days, step on the scales now and write in your weight in the space underneath the picture. Be sure to fill in today's date as well.

As soon as you've done these three things, you are ready to begin the transformation of a lifetime . . .

YOUR SUCCESS CALENDAR

START DATE .... **FINISH DATE** ....

1	2	3	4	5	6
7	8	9	10	11	12
13	14	**15**	16	17	18
19	20	21	22	23	24
25	26	27	28	29	**30**
31	32	33	34	35	36
37	38	39	40	41	42
43	44	**45**	46	47	48
49	50	51	52	53	54
55	56	57	58	59	**60**
61	62	63	64	65	66
67	68	69	70	71	72
73	74	**75**	76	77	78
79	80	81	82	83	84
85	86	87	88	89	**90**

Cross each day off your success calendar as you work through the programme . . .

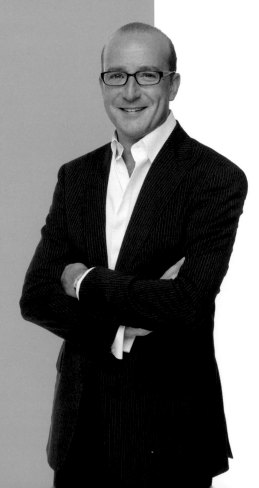

> **THE GREATEST THING IN THIS WORLD IS NOT SO MUCH WHERE WE STAND AS IN WHAT DIRECTION WE ARE MOVING.**
>
> JOHANN WOLFGANG VON GOETHE

WEEK 1

STARTING STRONG!

DAY 01

BEGIN WITH THE END IN MIND

Today, it begins – the first day of what will probably be an entirely new relationship with food and an entirely new relationship with your body. But where will it all end?

Take a few moments to do the following:

Close your eyes and imagine that it's 90 days from today. If it helps, mark the date on a real or imaginary calendar. Now travel out into the future until you are looking at a future, slimmer, happier you. When you're ready, step into that future you until you're seeing what they see, hearing what they hear, and feeling the wonderful feelings in your brand new body.

The more you allow yourself to really enjoy this feeling, the easier it will be to return to this visualization again and again throughout the 90 days – and every time you do, you are programming your mind for success!

> **START BY DOING WHAT'S NECESSARY; THEN DO WHAT'S POSSIBLE; AND SUDDENLY YOU ARE DOING THE IMPOSSIBLE.**
> ST FRANCIS OF ASSISI

TODAY'S SUCCESS CHECKLIST

- [1] I ate when I was hungry
- [2] I ate what I really wanted
- [3] I ate consciously
- [4] I stopped when full
- [5] I drank water
- [6] I moved my body
- [7] I listened to the CD
- [8] I did the mirror exercise

One **Positive Thing** I Noticed Today . . .

What I'm **Looking Forward To** Tomorrow . . .

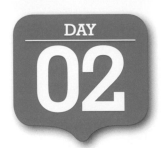

A PICTURE OF SUCCESS

**THE HUMAN BODY
IS THE BEST PICTURE
OF THE HUMAN SOUL.**

LUDWIG WITTGENSTEIN

Have you ever seen one of those pictures of an athlete in the moment of victory? Even as we look at another person reaching their goal, our own resolve and will to win is strengthened.

Today, take some time to find a picture of something or someone that inspires you. Put it up somewhere where you'll see it every day (such as the refrigerator!) or carry it around in your purse, wallet or even inside this book. Whenever you need an extra dose of courage or determination, you can look at the picture and inspire yourself to success!

TODAY'S SUCCESS CHECKLIST

1. I ate when I was hungry
2. I ate what I really wanted
3. I ate consciously
4. I stopped when full
5. I drank water
6. I moved my body
7. I listened to the CD
8. I did the mirror exercise

One **Positive Thing** I Noticed Today . . .

What I'm **Looking Forward To** Tomorrow . . .

DAY
03

EMPTY YOUR REFRIGERATOR

You may have, in the past, been on one diet or another that told you to empty your cupboards of any foods high in fat, sugar, carbohydrates, or whatever food you were being forbidden to eat.

My instructions for you are radically different.

Today, I want you to go into your refrigerator and throw out any food that does not totally inspire you to eat it. Chuck the diet drinks. Throw out the low-fat yogurts. Unless you love them, bin the sugar-free popsicles. You'll know that you're done when there isn't a single thing in your fridge that you wouldn't be delighted to eat – and when you're next hungry, that's exactly what I'm asking you to do!

> **PART OF THE SECRET OF SUCCESS IN LIFE IS TO EAT WHAT YOU LIKE AND LET THE FOOD FIGHT IT OUT INSIDE.**
> MARK TWAIN

TODAY'S SUCCESS CHECKLIST

- [ ] 1   I ate when I was hungry
- [ ] 2   I ate what I really wanted
- [ ] 3   I ate consciously
- [ ] 4   I stopped when full
- [ ] 5   I drank water
- [ ] 6   I moved my body
- [ ] 7   I listened to the CD
- [ ] 8   I did the mirror exercise

One **Positive Thing** I Noticed Today . . .

What I'm **Looking Forward To** Tomorrow . . .

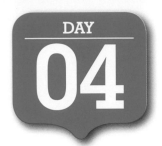

DAY 04

ACCEPT YOURSELF!

When we focus on our goals for the future, it can sometimes seem as though we are really rejecting who we are in the present.

Take a few minutes to stand in front of the mirror today and send love and approval to your body. Remember, acceptance doesn't mean that you don't want to change something – it just means that you are willing to accept that where you are now is where you are now.

> **EVERYTHING IN LIFE THAT WE REALLY ACCEPT UNDERGOES A CHANGE.**
> KATHERINE MANSFIELD

TODAY'S SUCCESS CHECKLIST

1 I ate when I was hungry

2 I ate what I really wanted

3 I ate consciously

4 I stopped when full

5 I drank water

6 I moved my body

7 I listened to the CD

8 I did the mirror exercise

One **Positive Thing** I Noticed Today . . .

....

....

What I'm **Looking Forward To** Tomorrow . . .

....

....

DAY 05

THE BEST YEAR OF YOUR LIFE

Chances are that if you're using this journal, you've already decided that it's time for a change. But you may not yet realize that you're probably thinking too small . . .

> **YOU WILL THINK MORE THAN 50,000 THOUGHTS TODAY, SO YOU MIGHT AS WELL MAKE THEM BIG ONES!**
> DONALD TRUMP

Close your eyes and vividly imagine it's a year from now and you have had your best year so far. What must have happened for that to be true? Be specific about each area of your life:

- **My health**
- **My career**
- **My relationships**
- **My finances**
- **My spirituality**

Remember it's important to be clear. If you put vagueness out, you will get vague results back. So take a few minutes and imagine your life has become outrageously better. Then at least five times today, spend a few moments thinking about how good your life can be!

TODAY'S SUCCESS CHECKLIST

1. I ate when I was hungry

2. I ate what I really wanted

3. I ate consciously

4. I stopped when full

5. I drank water

6. I moved my body

7. I listened to the CD

8. I did the mirror exercise

One **Positive Thing** I Noticed Today . . .

What I'm **Looking Forward To** Tomorrow . . .

TODAY'S SUCCESS CHECKLIST

☐ 1 I ate when I was hungry

☐ 2 I ate what I really wanted

☐ 3 I ate consciously

☐ 4 I stopped when full

☐ 5 I drank water

☐ 6 I moved my body

☐ 7 I listened to the CD

☐ 8 I did the mirror exercise

One **Positive Thing**
I Noticed Today . . .

....

....

....

What I'm **Looking Forward To**
Tomorrow . . .

....

....

....

....

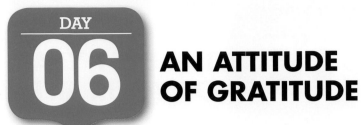

AN ATTITUDE OF GRATITUDE

When we are wrapped up in our own worries and concerns, it is the easiest thing in the world to overlook all the good things we already have in our lives.

Today, we are going to reverse that pattern by asking yourself to focus on what's already working well in your life. Ask and answer these questions each time you notice you are hungry. When you've fed your heart, it will be time to feed your body . . .

- **Who do I love?**
- **Who loves me?**
- **What am I most grateful for in my life?**
- **What is it about that which makes me feel grateful?**

> **FEELING GRATITUDE AND NOT EXPRESSING IT IS LIKE WRAPPING A PRESENT AND NOT GIVING IT.**
>
> WILLIAM ARTHUR WARD

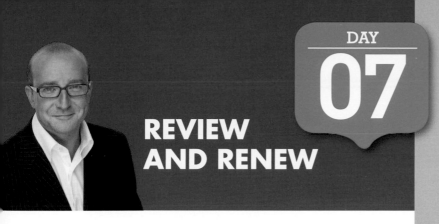

REVIEW AND RENEW

HOPE IS A RENEWABLE OPTION: IF YOU RUN OUT OF IT AT THE END OF THE DAY, YOU GET TO START OVER IN THE MORNING.

BARBARA KINGSOLVER

Every seven days, I'm going to ask you to take time out to reflect on how far you've come and refocus on where you are heading. Here's your very first chance to 'review and renew' . . .

1. The best things that happened this week were:

....

2. My biggest challenges this week were:

....

3. I did these things for the first time:

....

4. What I learned was:

....

5. My top three priorities for the week ahead are:

a.
....

b.
....

c.
....

TODAY'S SUCCESS CHECKLIST

☐ 1 I ate when I was hungry

☐ 2 I ate what I really wanted

☐ 3 I ate consciously

☐ 4 I stopped when full

☐ 5 I drank water

☐ 6 I moved my body

☐ 7 I listened to the CD

☐ 8 I did the mirror exercise

One **Positive Thing** I Noticed Today . . .

....

....

What I'm **Looking Forward To** Tomorrow . . .

....

....

....

> **SIMPLICITY IS THE ULTIMATE SOPHISTICATION.**
> LEONARDO DA VINCI

THE FOUR GOLDEN RULES

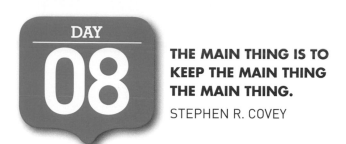

**THE MAIN THING IS TO
KEEP THE MAIN THING
THE MAIN THING.**
STEPHEN R. COVEY

THE FOUR GOLDEN RULES TO LOSING WEIGHT FOR EVER

This week, we'll go through each of the golden rules to success again and reinforce them as habits. For today, just imagine what it would be like to really eat this way:

Imagine yourself tuning in to your body and noticing you're a little bit hungry. In the past, you might have ignored this sensation, but now you've learned to respect it. You ask your body what it wants and needs. To your amazement, it asks for a small bowl of pasta with a salad. (You were sure it was going to be chocolate cake and ice cream, weren't you?) Resisting the urge to skip the pasta, you sit down for a wonderful, peaceful meal. Stopping to smell your food between each mouthful, you enjoy indulging in the sensation of the warm pasta melting in your mouth before sliding easily down your throat. Each bite of salad crunches in your mouth, and you can taste the water-rich juice from the lettuce and cucumber with every mouthful. Delicious!

Down towards the bottom of the bowl, you realize you are comfortably full. Imagine the sense of pride as you push away the rest of the bowl, knowing that you are now in full control . . .

TODAY'S SUCCESS CHECKLIST

1. ☐ I ate when I was hungry

2. ☐ I ate what I really wanted

3. ☐ I ate consciously

4. ☐ I stopped when full

5. ☐ I drank water

6. ☐ I moved my body

7. ☐ I listened to the CD

8. ☐ I did the mirror exercise

One **Positive Thing**
I Noticed Today . . .

What I'm **Looking Forward To**
Tomorrow . . .

155

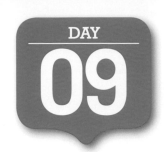

RULE 1: WHEN YOU ARE HUNGRY, EAT

ONCE YOU LEARN TO QUIT, IT BECOMES A HABIT.

VINCENT LOMBARDI

I was amazed when someone told me she was shocked to hear that one of the keys to losing weight and keeping it off was to eat when she was hungry.

'If I did that,' she told me, 'I'd never stop.'

Isn't it funny how some people are such experts on what they've never done? It's time to end the self-inflicted torture and listen to your body instead!

Make this commitment:

'I, _____, promise that for at least the next 81 days, I will eat whenever I'm hungry no matter how I feel about it.'

TODAY'S SUCCESS CHECKLIST

1. I ate when I was hungry
2. I ate what I really wanted
3. I ate consciously
4. I stopped when full
5. I drank water
6. I moved my body
7. I listened to the CD
8. I did the mirror exercise

One **Positive Thing** I Noticed Today . . .

What I'm **Looking Forward To** Tomorrow . . .

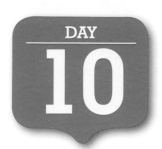

DAY 10

RULE 2: EAT WHAT YOU WANT, NOT WHAT YOU THINK YOU SHOULD

There are NO forbidden foods in my system – you can eat anything you want any time you are hungry, providing you take the time to really, really enjoy eating it.

Fancy a bit of pasta? Go for it.

Cake and ice cream calling to you? As long as you're actually hungry, enjoy, enjoy, enjoy.

From this day forward, nothing is off-limits to you. Ever.

And if you still really want to say 'NO' to something, say it to the purveyors of sugar-free low-carb cardboard-tasting crap.

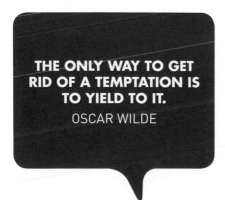

THE ONLY WAY TO GET RID OF A TEMPTATION IS TO YIELD TO IT.
OSCAR WILDE

1. ☐ I ate when I was hungry

2. ☐ I ate what I really wanted

3. ☐ I ate consciously

4. ☐ I stopped when full

5. ☐ I drank water

6. ☐ I moved my body

7. ☐ I listened to the CD

8. ☐ I did the mirror exercise

One **Positive Thing**
I Noticed Today . . .

What I'm **Looking Forward To**
Tomorrow . . .

- [1] I ate when I was hungry

- [2] I ate what I really wanted

- [3] I ate consciously

- [4] I stopped when full

- [5] I drank water

- [6] I moved my body

- [7] I listened to the CD

- [8] I did the mirror exercise

One **Positive Thing**
I Noticed Today . . .

What I'm **Looking Forward To**
Tomorrow . . .

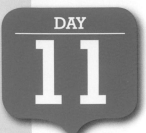

DAY 11

PLEASURE IS THE OBJECT, THE DUTY AND THE GOAL OF ALL RATIONAL CREATURES.

VOLTAIRE

RULE 3: EAT CONSCIOUSLY AND ENJOY EVERY MOUTHFUL

Here's an experiment for you to try today:

1 Create a 'sample platter' with a taste of each of your favourite foods: a bit of warm bread with butter, a slice of sharp cheddar cheese, a bite of a bar of chocolate, a bit of sushi – anything that makes your mouth water just thinking about it.

2 Indulge your senses. Close your eyes and smell your food before eating it. See how long you can make each bite last. Pay close attention and notice flavours and textures changing as you chew. Food has many tastes if you take the time to savour it.

3 Notice which foods become more enjoyable the longer you take to eat them, and any that may become less enjoyable. Try to discover at least one new flavour in each food you sample.

Remember, the more you are willing to enjoy each mouthful, the thinner you are becoming!

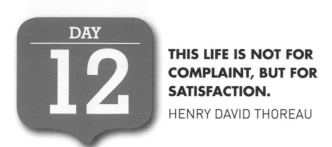

THIS LIFE IS NOT FOR COMPLAINT, BUT FOR SATISFACTION.

HENRY DAVID THOREAU

RULE 4: WHEN YOU THINK YOU ARE FULL, STOP EATING

What's the first sign for you that your body is getting full and satisfied with what you've eaten?

Here are what some of the people on my seminars have said:

I know I'm getting full when my stomach starts to grumble.

I know I'm getting full when the food stops tasting quite so good.

I know I'm getting full when I can't think of anything else I'd like to eat.

I know I'm getting full because I suspect I might be.

What is it for you?

If you're not sure, take some time today to really tune into your body as you eat and notice what the very first sign of satisfaction and fullness is for you. The more aware of your body's signals you become, the easier it will be for you to not only lose those extra pounds but to keep them off for good!

TODAY'S SUCCESS CHECKLIST

1. I ate when I was hungry

2. I ate what I really wanted

3. I ate consciously

4. I stopped when full

5. I drank water

6. I moved my body

7. I listened to the CD

8. I did the mirror exercise

One **Positive Thing** I Noticed Today . . .

What I'm **Looking Forward To** Tomorrow . . .

159

TODAY'S SUCCESS CHECKLIST

1. ☐ I ate when I was hungry

2. ☐ I ate what I really wanted

3. ☐ I ate consciously

4. ☐ I stopped when full

5. ☐ I drank water

6. ☐ I moved my body

7. ☐ I listened to the CD

8. ☐ I did the mirror exercise

One **Positive Thing**
I Noticed Today . . .

....

....

....

What I'm **Looking Forward To**
Tomorrow . . .

....

....

....

....

....

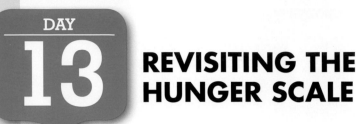

REVISITING THE HUNGER SCALE

Perhaps the most useful tool you can use in your quest for more pleasure and less weight is the **Hunger Scale:**

1. Physically faint
2. Ravenous
3. **Fairly hungry**
4. **Slightly hungry**
5. **Neutral**
6. **Pleasantly satisfied**
7. Full
8. Stuffed
9. Bloated
10. Nauseous

Remember, ideally you want to begin eating between 3 and 4 and finish eating around 6. The more you go to one extreme, the more likely you are to go to the other. By avoiding both extremes, you will be living your life in balance.

> **LIVING IN BALANCE AND PURITY IS THE HIGHEST GOOD FOR YOU AND THE EARTH.**
>
> DEEPAK CHOPRA

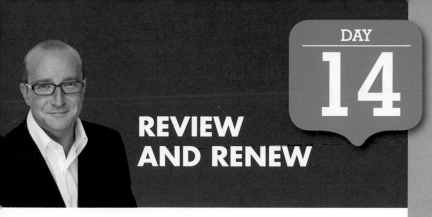

DAY 14

REVIEW AND RENEW

THE MORE YOU PRAISE AND CELEBRATE YOUR LIFE, THE MORE THERE IS IN LIFE TO CELEBRATE.

OPRAH WINFREY

You're two weeks in to a brand new way of eating – how does it feel? Exciting? Scary? Both?

Prepare for tomorrow today by taking some time to review and renew . . .

1. The best things that happened this week were:

....

2. My biggest challenges this week were:

....

3. I did these things for the first time:

....

4. What I learned was:

....

5. My top three priorities for the week ahead are:

a. ....

b. ....

c. ....

TODAY'S SUCCESS CHECKLIST

1 I ate when I was hungry

2 I ate what I really wanted

3 I ate consciously

4 I stopped when full

5 I drank water

6 I moved my body

7 I listened to the CD

8 I did the mirror exercise

One **Positive Thing** I Noticed Today . . .

....

....

What I'm **Looking Forward To** Tomorrow . . .

....

....

....

> YOU HAVE TO EAT
> REGULARLY TO MAINTAIN
> YOUR ENERGY LEVELS
> – IF YOU STARVE YOUR
> BODY, IT SIMPLY STORES
> EVERYTHING THAT
> YOU DO EAT.
>
> CINDY CRAWFORD

YOUR FIRST CHECK-IN . . .

Congratulations! For two weeks now, you have been interrupting your old patterns of diet and exercise and building the foundations for a whole new way or relating to food, your emotions and your body. By the time you are finished with this journal, it will be as difficult for you to go back to your old way of doing things as it will be easy and natural to eat and live in a way that truly works for you.

Remember, this journal is designed to support you in creating the habits of empowered eating.

Take a moment now to jot down anything you've already noticed about how things are changing . . .

....
....
....
....
....
....
....
....
....
....
....
....

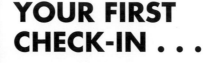

TODAY I WEIGH

MANJIT SAHOTA

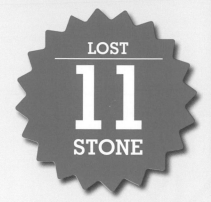

LOST
11
STONE

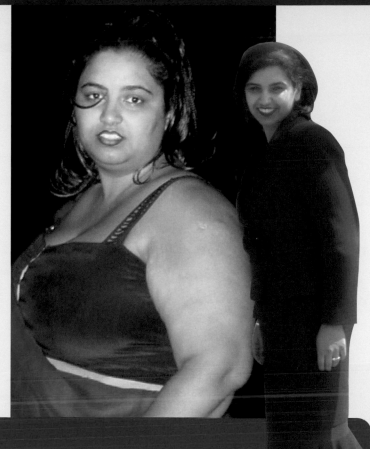

MANJIT'S STORY

I'd always been overweight. Since early childhood I'd been on every diet you could think of. After seeing my honeymoon pictures, I was distraught. That same week I saw Paul's book and started reading it at once. For a week, I followed the instructions and listened to the CD.

Something just clicked. I made losing weight into an objective and my mind was set. I've never been able to lose so much weight so easily before . . . and enjoy everything I was doing to achieve it!

I cannot overemphasize the value of the tools and techniques – and the fun I had reading the book. I continue to use the tools and technique in other aspects of my life, too, with many positive outcomes. I can simply say that this does what it says on the packet. The techniques in this book changed my life and made my dreams come true.

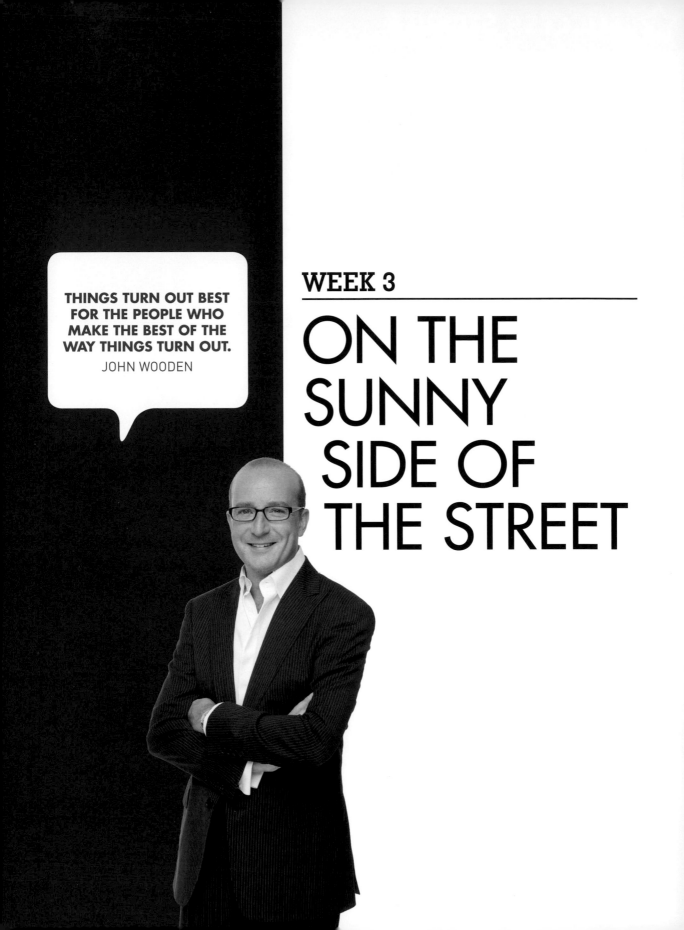

THINGS TURN OUT BEST
FOR THE PEOPLE WHO
MAKE THE BEST OF THE
WAY THINGS TURN OUT.

JOHN WOODEN

WEEK 3

ON THE
SUNNY
SIDE OF
THE STREET

THE SECRET OF STAYING YOUNG IS TO LIVE HONESTLY, EAT SLOWLY, AND LIE ABOUT YOUR AGE. LUCILLE BALL

One of my favourites of the exercises we do on our NLP trainings is called 'On the Sunny Side of the Street'. In groups of five or six people, someone calls out something that would generally be thought of as negative. Everyone in the group then has to come up with a way in which that could be perceived as a positive. For example, if somebody said, 'I think about food all the time', people in the group might respond:

> 'You must be an expert by now – maybe you could host a talk show!'

> 'Wow – I bet that means you're a very sensual person!'

> 'At least you can think!'

The purpose of the exercise is not to convince yourself to be happy about something you're not, but rather to recognize and increase your capacity to find the positive in the midst of a challenge.

Have a go right now . . .

1 Think of something you're a little bit unhappy about in your life.

2 Come up with at least three ways it could be seen as a good thing – the more outrageous the better!

TODAY'S SUCCESS CHECKLIST

- [1] I ate when I was hungry
- [2] I ate what I really wanted
- [3] I ate consciously
- [4] I stopped when full
- [5] I drank water
- [6] I moved my body
- [7] I listened to the CD
- [8] I did the mirror exercise

One **Positive Thing** I Noticed Today . . .

What I'm **Looking Forward To** Tomorrow . . .

1 ☐ I ate when I was hungry

2 ☐ I ate what I really wanted

3 ☐ I ate consciously

4 ☐ I stopped when full

5 ☐ I drank water

6 ☐ I moved my body

7 ☐ I listened to the CD

8 ☐ I did the mirror exercise

One **Positive Thing**
I Noticed Today . . .

What I'm **Looking Forward To**
Tomorrow . . .

DAY 17
ELIMINATE THE NEGATIVE

Over the years, I have worked with any number of struggling actors and musicians who resented the rich and famous while simultaneously striving to join their ranks. The problem with that is simple:

It's difficult to become something if you hate it.

Your unconscious mind craves consistency – and if you keep telling it that you hate all naturally thin people, it will do whatever it can not to let you become one of them.

There is something miraculously freeing about celebrating the success of others, even those people we don't particularly like. Try it as an experiment for the next few days. Whenever you hear about someone doing well, think something congratulatory. Bless their success instead of cursing it. Shortly this will become a new habit and you will become a more positive person.

And as you begin to wish the best for those who are thinner than you, your unconscious mind will begin to make you more like them!

> **BETTER TO LIGHT A CANDLE THAN TO CURSE THE DARKNESS.**
> CHINESE PROVERB

DAY 18

APPROVAL, APPROVAL, APPROVAL, APPROVAL, APPROVAL

A MAN CANNOT BE COMFORTABLE WITHOUT HIS OWN APPROVAL.

MARK TWAIN

A lady came on one of my easy-weight-loss seminars determined that this time things would be different. Whatever the programme was, she was going to follow it to the letter until she'd lost every pound she'd packed on since her last baby was born. But when I asked her to look in the mirror and approve of herself as she was, she wanted to leave the room.

'I've never approved of myself,' she confessed. 'I'm not sure I know how.'

Here is all that you need to do:

1 Begin by sending approval to your big toe, or any part of your body about which you are indifferent. Simply tell it that you approve of it and are willing to love it as it is right now.

2 Work your way through every part of your body until you can love and approve of EVERYTHING. If you've really never done this before, it's OK if it takes a few days or even weeks.

Remember, approval doesn't mean you won't change – it just means you won't be in terrible emotional pain while you do!

TODAY'S SUCCESS CHECKLIST

1 I ate when I was hungry

2 I ate what I really wanted

3 I ate consciously

4 I stopped when full

5 I drank water

6 I moved my body

7 I listened to the CD

8 I did the mirror exercise

One **Positive Thing** I Noticed Today . . .

What I'm **Looking Forward To** Tomorrow . . .

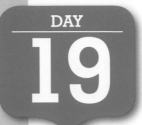
FAILURE IS A FEW ERRORS IN JUDGEMENT, REPEATED EVERY DAY.

JIM ROHN

TODAY'S SUCCESS CHECKLIST

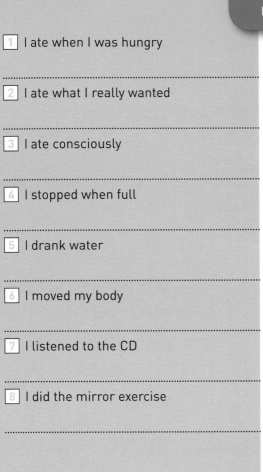

1 I ate when I was hungry

2 I ate what I really wanted

3 I ate consciously

4 I stopped when full

5 I drank water

6 I moved my body

7 I listened to the CD

8 I did the mirror exercise

One **Positive Thing**
I Noticed Today . . .

What I'm **Looking Forward To**
Tomorrow . . .

PULL YOURSELF OUT OF THE STREAM OF JUDGEMENTS

If you ever tune into the stream of judgements running through your mind during the course of the day, you could be excused for thinking you were going to drown.

> 'Oh my god, look at those thighs!'
>
> 'Does she really think he's going to look twice at her in that dress?'
>
> 'I'm fat. Horrible and fat. Horrible, ugly, miserable and fat.'

The truth is, nearly everyone has a stream of thoughts going on in their head all day long, and if they're not careful, they can start to get stuck inside their own minds.

Today, whenever you meet someone, talk with them or even pass them by in the street, silently say the word 'Peace'. If your brain has been chattering away, it will suddenly go quiet and bring you back into the present moment.

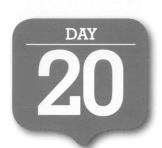

WHAT YOU PRACTISE, YOU BECOME

ALWAYS ACT AS IF YOU HAVE ALREADY ACHIEVED WHAT IT IS YOU ARE SETTING OUT TO ACCOMPLISH.

JOE D. BATTEN

How do you think you'll be different when you've lost the weight you want to lose? Will you be happier? Have more energy? Feel better about yourself?

While all these things are possible, they become more likely when you begin to practise them even before you've lost the weight. Want to be happy, energized and filled with positive self-regard?

Then practise, practise, practise!

TODAY'S SUCCESS CHECKLIST

1   I ate when I was hungry

2   I ate what I really wanted

3   I ate consciously

4   I stopped when full

5   I drank water

6   I moved my body

7   I listened to the CD

8   I did the mirror exercise

One **Positive Thing** I Noticed Today . . .

What I'm **Looking Forward To** Tomorrow . . .

1 I ate when I was hungry

2 I ate what I really wanted

3 I ate consciously

4 I stopped when full

5 I drank water

6 I moved my body

7 I listened to the CD

8 I did the mirror exercise

One **Positive Thing**
I Noticed Today . . .

What I'm **Looking Forward To**
Tomorrow . . .

DAY
21 SEE YOURSELF SLIM

Just as athletes rehearse success in their minds over and over again, you need to imagine exactly how you will be when you are thinner. By constantly thinking about how you ultimately want to look, you are programming your mind to make you more and more that way.

Do this simple exercise several times today:

1 Imagine how good you will look when you are a little bit thinner than you are right now.

2 Float into that thinner you. See through their eyes, hear through their ears and feel how good it feels.

3 Now, imagine how good you will look when you are a little bit thinner than that.

4 Once again, float into that thinner you and enjoy the experience.

5 Keep doing this until you can easily imagine being your ideal weight. The more you do it, the easier it becomes.

> **VISUALIZATION IS DAYDREAMING WITH A PURPOSE.**
> BO BENNETT

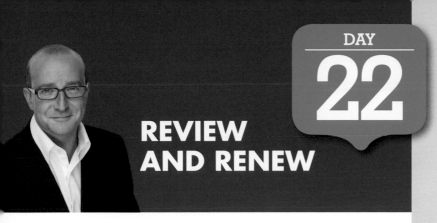

REVIEW AND RENEW

TODAY'S SUCCESS CHECKLIST

- **1** I ate when I was hungry
- **2** I ate what I really wanted
- **3** I ate consciously
- **4** I stopped when full
- **5** I drank water
- **6** I moved my body
- **7** I listened to the CD
- **8** I did the mirror exercise

One Positive Thing
I Noticed Today . . .

What I'm Looking Forward To
Tomorrow . . .

LEARN FROM YESTERDAY, LIVE FOR TODAY, HOPE FOR TOMORROW.

ALBERT EINSTEIN

You are now three weeks into this success journal, and the fact that you are still going means you really are making changes, inside and out. It's time once again to reflect on how far you've come and refocus on where you're heading.

1. The best things that happened this week were:

2. My biggest challenges this week were:

3. I did these things for the first time:

4. What I learned was:

5. My top three priorities for the week ahead are:

a.

b.

c.

> **THE BODY NEVER LIES.**
> MARTHA GRAHAM

LISTEN TO YOUR BODY!

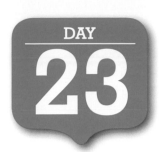

GETTING TO KNOW YOUR BODY

I THINK AWARENESS IS PROBABLY THE MOST IMPORTANT THING IN BECOMING A CHAMPION.

BILLIE JEAN KING

What's going on with your body right now? Take a minute now to do a complete inner body scan from head to toe (and yes, that does include 'stomach'!) . . .

Which parts of your body feel particularly good? Are there any parts of your body that are uncomfortable? Is there any part of your body that is 'unavailable' – i.e. that you can't get a sense of with your eyes closed?

Repeat this exercise at least three times today – make an effort to notice at least one new thing each time. As you become more aware of what's going on with your body throughout the day, it will become easier and easier to stay aware of what's going on with your body while you eat!

TODAY'S SUCCESS CHECKLIST

1. I ate when I was hungry

2. I ate what I really wanted

3. I ate consciously

4. I stopped when full

5. I drank water

6. I moved my body

7. I listened to the CD

8. I did the mirror exercise

One **Positive Thing** I Noticed Today . . .

What I'm **Looking Forward To** Tomorrow . . .

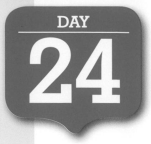
THE ONLY REASON I WOULD TAKE UP JOGGING IS SO THAT I COULD HEAR HEAVY BREATHING AGAIN.
ERMA BOMBECK

TODAY'S SUCCESS CHECKLIST

1 I ate when I was hungry

2 I ate what I really wanted

3 I ate consciously

4 I stopped when full

5 I drank water

6 I moved my body

7 I listened to the CD

8 I did the mirror exercise

One **Positive Thing** I Noticed Today . . .

What I'm **Looking Forward To** Tomorrow . . .

BREATHE MORE, EAT LESS

Given that people can go on a hunger strike for 90 days or more without dying, it's probably a bit of an exaggeration to say 'I'm starving' two hours after a Chinese takeaway. But the body can't survive even five minutes without a healthy supply of oxygen. And when you give the body the oxygen it craves, it will give you more energy and a faster metabolism.

Doing this simple breathing exercise before each meal is an excellent way of making sure you're giving your body what it really needs:

1 Breathe in through your nose for a count of 5.

2 Hold your breath for a count of 20. If you can't get to 20, just hold it as long as you can. Imagine pumping the oxygen through to every cell in your body, giving it the nourishment it truly wants and needs.

3 Now, exhale completely until your body is empty. Stay 'empty' for as long as you can.

4 When your body really wants to breathe in again, let it. Allow your breathing to return to normal.

5 Repeat at least two more times.

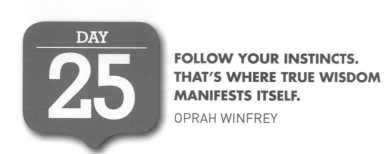

FOLLOW YOUR INSTINCTS. THAT'S WHERE TRUE WISDOM MANIFESTS ITSELF.

OPRAH WINFREY

HONOURING INNER WISDOM

If your body could talk, what would it say to you? Would it thank you for how lovingly you've been treating it, or would it shrink away like Oliver Twist, afraid to ask you for more? Throughout the day today, ask your body this question:

'What can I do to take better care of you in this moment?'

Regardless of whether the answer is 'take a deep breath', 'love me', or 'give me a cream cake!', honour your body's wisdom and do what you can to take care of it.

TODAY'S SUCCESS CHECKLIST

1. ☐ I ate when I was hungry

2. ☐ I ate what I really wanted

3. ☐ I ate consciously

4. ☐ I stopped when full

5. ☐ I drank water

6. ☐ I moved my body

7. ☐ I listened to the CD

8. ☐ I did the mirror exercise

One **Positive Thing** I Noticed Today . . .

....

....

What I'm **Looking Forward To** Tomorrow . . .

....

....

....

175

1. I ate when I was hungry

2. I ate what I really wanted

3. I ate consciously

4. I stopped when full

5. I drank water

6. I moved my body

7. I listened to the CD

8. I did the mirror exercise

One **Positive Thing**
I Noticed Today . . .

What I'm **Looking Forward To**
Tomorrow . . .

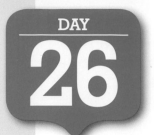

DAY 26

WATER ITS LIVING STRENGTH FIRST SHOWS, WHEN OBSTACLES ITS COURSE OPPOSE.
JOHANN WOLFGANG VON GOETHE

ARE YOU THIRSTY?

Did you know that when you feel hungry, there is a 75 per cent chance you are actually dehydrated? This is why one of the most valuable things you can do is to make sure you have a fresh glass of water before sitting down to eat.

One woman who lost 3 stone using my system credited the majority of the weight loss to this one distinction. As she said, 'I had always heard that it was healthy to drink at least eight glasses of water a day, but I could never get myself to do it. By simply drinking a glass of water before eating, I've increased my water intake effortlessly. After doing it for a few weeks, I realized how often I'd been misinterpreting my body's need for water as hunger for food. I now eat much less than I used to, but I never feel like I'm denying myself anything. And when I am hungry, I make sure to eat what I love and love eating it!'

Make a commitment right now to make sure you always have easy access to filtered or distilled water and to drink a glass every time before you eat. You'll be glad you did!

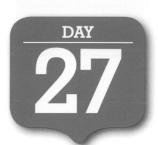

DAY 27

LOVE THE MOMENT, AND THE ENERGY OF THE MOMENT WILL SPREAD BEYOND ALL BOUNDARIES.

SISTER CORITA KENT

FOOD AS FUEL

There are two types of energy – potential and kinetic. Petrol is an example of potential energy – in and of itself, it just sits there, but when you stick it in an engine, it becomes 'kinetic' – it fuels the engine to take the car wherever you want to go. As the potential energy becomes kinetic, it gets used up and needs to be replenished.

Similarly, food is potential energy for the engine of your body. This is why it's so important to eat when you're hungry and to move your body.

If you kept driving without putting in enough petrol, what would you expect to happen to your engine? It would continually splutter and stall, and eventually wear out. On the other hand, if you kept putting petrol into a car without ever driving it, the petrol would begin overflowing everywhere, creating a safety hazard and a bit of a mess.

By balancing eating when you're hungry (filling the tank) and moving your body frequently (driving the car), your body will reward you by taking you wherever you want to go!

TODAY'S SUCCESS CHECKLIST

1. ☐ I ate when I was hungry

2. ☐ I ate what I really wanted

3. ☐ I ate consciously

4. ☐ I stopped when full

5. ☐ I drank water

6. ☐ I moved my body

7. ☐ I listened to the CD

8. ☐ I did the mirror exercise

One **Positive Thing** I Noticed Today . . .

....

....

What I'm **Looking Forward To** Tomorrow . . .

....

....

....

1 I ate when I was hungry

2 I ate what I really wanted

3 I ate consciously

4 I stopped when full

5 I drank water

6 I moved my body

7 I listened to the CD

8 I did the mirror exercise

One **Positive Thing**
I Noticed Today . . .

What I'm **Looking Forward To**
Tomorrow . . .

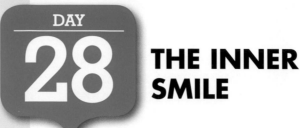

DAY 28
THE INNER SMILE

Here is one of my favourite exercises from **Change Your Life in 7 Days:**

1 Sit comfortably – ultimately, you can practise the inner smile anywhere in any position.

2 Allow a smile to dance into your eyes. If you like, raise the corner of your mouth ever so slightly, like someone who knows a really good secret but isn't going to tell.

3 Smile into any part of your body that feels tight or uncomfortable until it begins to ease or relax.

4 Smile into any part of your body that feels especially good. You can increase the smile by expressing gratitude to that part of your body for helping to keep you healthy and strong.

5 Allow the inner smile to reach every nook and cranny of your body.

> **A SMILE IS A CURVE THAT SETS EVERYTHING STRAIGHT.**
> PHYLLIS DILLER

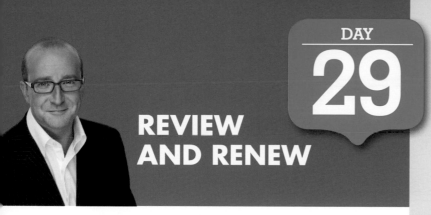

REVIEW AND RENEW

TODAY'S SUCCESS CHECKLIST

- [1] I ate when I was hungry
- [2] I ate what I really wanted
- [3] I ate consciously
- [4] I stopped when full
- [5] I drank water
- [6] I moved my body
- [7] I listened to the CD
- [8] I did the mirror exercise

IF YOU WATCH HOW NATURE DEALS WITH ADVERSITY, CONTINUALLY RENEWING ITSELF, YOU CANNOT HELP BUT LEARN.

BERNIE S. SIEGEL

As you continue changing your eating habits day by day and week by week, it's important to step back from time to time and see how far you've already come. Take a few moments now to learn from the wisdom of your own experience . . .

1. The best things that happened this week were:

....

2. My biggest challenges this week were:

....

3. I did these things for the first time:

....

4. What I learned was:

....

5. My top three priorities for the week ahead are:

a. ....

b. ....

c. ....

One **Positive Thing**
I Noticed Today . . .

....

....

What I'm **Looking Forward To**
Tomorrow . . .

....

....

....

179

DAY 30

> SUCCESS IS NEITHER MAGICAL NOR MYSTERIOUS. SUCCESS IS THE NATURAL CONSEQUENCE OF CONSISTENTLY APPLYING THE BASIC FUNDAMENTALS.
>
> JIM ROHN

YOUR SECOND CHECK-IN . . .

I have to say I'm impressed. The fact that you've come this far is proof that you have what it takes to change your relationship with food forever. You've probably already begun to notice changes in your energy levels and maybe even your clothes size.

Take some time today to reflect on how things have already begun to change for the better . . .

....

....

....

....

....

....

....

....

....

....

....

....

....

....

TODAY I WEIGH

MICHAEL GEE

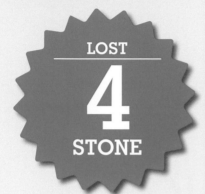

LOST
4
STONE

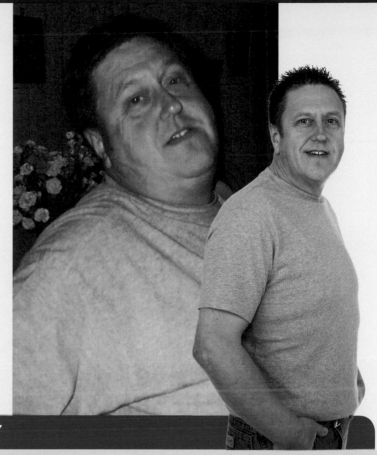

MICHAEL'S STORY

I had struggled with my weight all my life. A few years ago I was diagnosed with type-2 diabetes, mainly because of being obese, and I was put on medication.

I joined a gym and started swimming five mornings a week, which helped my blood sugar level but had no real impact on my obesity. I heard about Paul's weight-loss programme and attended a seminar in January 2005. By September 2005 I'd lost over 4 stone! It's so easy to lose weight it's immoral.

My family and friends say I look great, ten years younger, but the best thing is that I feel twenty years younger. My GP has reduced my medication and I believe I will soon be off medication altogether. Also, the seminar was a fantastic day. I gained so much that day. I had never enjoyed anything like it and it changed my life forever.

> **MOTIVATION IS WHAT GETS YOU STARTED. HABIT IS WHAT KEEPS YOU GOING.**
>
> JIM RYUN

WEEK 5

KEEP GOING!

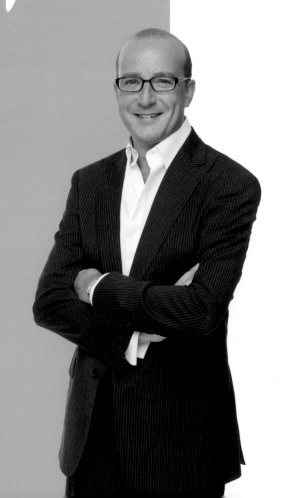

DAY 31

PRESS ON!

As you move into the second month of your 90-day success journal, it's important to keep your passion burning and your commitment alive.

One of my favourite 'power thoughts' on the value of persistence comes from former US president Calvin Coolidge:

'Nothing in the world can take the place of persistence. Talent will not; nothing is more common than unsuccessful men with talent. Genius will not; unrewarded genius is almost a proverb. Education will not; the world is full of educated derelicts. Persistence and determination alone are omnipotent. The slogan "Press on" has solved and always will solve the problems of the human race.'

Whether you're feeling excited or daunted as you look ahead, I have only one thing to say to you:

Press on!

> **YOU ALWAYS PASS FAILURE ON THE WAY TO SUCCESS.**
> MICKEY ROONEY

TODAY'S SUCCESS CHECKLIST

- [1] I ate when I was hungry
- [2] I ate what I really wanted
- [3] I ate consciously
- [4] I stopped when full
- [5] I drank water
- [6] I moved my body
- [7] I listened to the CD
- [8] I did the mirror exercise

One **Positive Thing** I Noticed Today . . .

What I'm **Looking Forward To** Tomorrow . . .

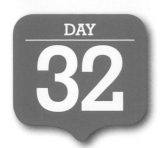

THE MOTIVATION BOOSTER!

PEOPLE OFTEN SAY THAT MOTIVATION DOESN'T LAST. WELL, NEITHER DOES BATHING – THAT'S WHY WE RECOMMEND IT DAILY.

ZIG ZIGLAR

Here's a simple exercise you can do any time you feel your motivation beginning to flag or your resolve weaken:

1 Make a list of all the reasons you don't want to be overweight.

2 Make a list of all the reasons you do want to be thin and optimally healthy.

3 Make a list of all the diets you've tried in the past and how long (or short) they lasted.

4 Finally, make a list of the best things you've learned and experienced so far in the process of enjoying eating what you really want when you're actually hungry and stopping when you're full!

TODAY'S SUCCESS CHECKLIST

1 I ate when I was hungry

2 I ate what I really wanted

3 I ate consciously

4 I stopped when full

5 I drank water

6 I moved my body

7 I listened to the CD

8 I did the mirror exercise

One **Positive Thing** I Noticed Today . . .

....

....

....

What I'm **Looking Forward To** Tomorrow . . .

....

....

....

CAUGHT IN THE ACT

Ken Blanchard, co-author of the bestselling **One-Minute Manager** books, was at one time a schoolteacher who instituted an unusual practice. Instead of trying to catch students misbehaving or breaking the rules, he would wander around the school seeking to 'catch' kids doing something right.

Today, catch yourself doing as many things 'right' as you possibly can. If you like, go out and buy some gold stars and give yourself one for everything you do well or in keeping with the standards you have set for yourself.

If you really want to make it a great day, catch the people around you doing things right and share your gold stars with them!

CELEBRATE WHAT YOU WANT TO SEE MORE OF.
TOM PETERS

TODAY'S SUCCESS CHECKLIST

1. I ate when I was hungry

2. I ate what I really wanted

3. I ate consciously

4. I stopped when full

5. I drank water

6. I moved my body

7. I listened to the CD

8. I did the mirror exercise

One **Positive Thing** I Noticed Today . . .

What I'm **Looking Forward To** Tomorrow . . .

WE DON'T STOP PLAYING BECAUSE WE GROW OLD; WE GROW OLD BECAUSE WE STOP PLAYING.

GEORGE BERNARD SHAW

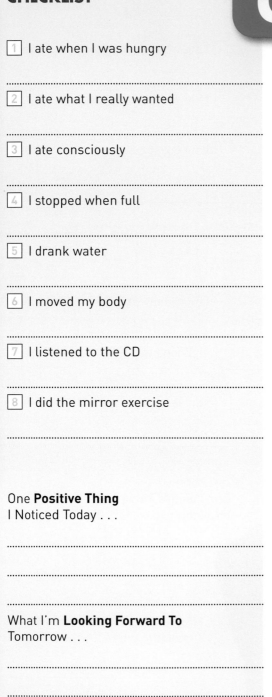

TODAY'S SUCCESS CHECKLIST

1. I ate when I was hungry

2. I ate what I really wanted

3. I ate consciously

4. I stopped when full

5. I drank water

6. I moved my body

7. I listened to the CD

8. I did the mirror exercise

One **Positive Thing** I Noticed Today . . .

What I'm **Looking Forward To** Tomorrow . . .

INCREASE THE 'FUN FACTOR'

One of the unsung rules of success is this:

What's fun gets done.

How can you make the process of using this journal and transforming your relationship with food even more fun?

Here are some of my favourite ideas from participants on my seminars:

Blow up 90 balloons and pop one for each day you successfully complete the programme.

Do the programme with a friend – cook great meals for one another, go for walks and share your successes.

Keep your eye on the prize – stick a photo of your head on your future body and enjoy the journey!

Jot down your own ideas here:

To make this programme even more fun, I could . . .

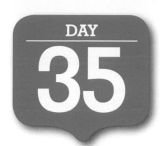

DANCE!

THOSE WHO DANCED WERE THOUGHT TO BE QUITE INSANE BY THOSE WHO COULD NOT HEAR THE MUSIC.

ANGELA MONET

Of all the ways you can move your body, enhance your metabolism and feel great, dancing is probably the most overlooked and most fun.

Today, put some vibrant music on and shake it like you just don't care – if you do this daily, there'll soon be a whole lot less of you to shake!

TODAY'S SUCCESS CHECKLIST

1. I ate when I was hungry
2. I ate what I really wanted
3. I ate consciously
4. I stopped when full
5. I drank water
6. I moved my body
7. I listened to the CD
8. I did the mirror exercise

One **Positive Thing** I Noticed Today . . .

What I'm **Looking Forward To** Tomorrow . . .

1. ☐ I ate when I was hungry

2. ☐ I ate what I really wanted

3. ☐ I ate consciously

4. ☐ I stopped when full

5. ☐ I drank water

6. ☐ I moved my body

7. ☐ I listened to the CD

8. ☐ I did the mirror exercise

One **Positive Thing**
I Noticed Today . . .

....

....

What I'm **Looking Forward To**
Tomorrow . . .

....

....

....

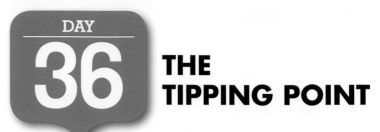

DAY 36
THE TIPPING POINT

There comes a point in the creation of any new habit where it becomes easier to do something than not do it. This is true whether the habit is a negative one (smoking or dieting) or a positive one (exercise, kindness, eating when you're hungry).

With each of the new habits you are creating through doing this programme, notice when you come to the 'tipping point' – that point where it has become easier to eat what you love than what you're supposed to, and when it becomes easier to stop when you're full than to stop when the plate is empty.

> **WE FIRST MAKE OUR HABITS, THEN OUR HABITS MAKE US.**
> JOHN DRYDEN

REVIEW AND RENEW

TODAY'S SUCCESS CHECKLIST

- **1** I ate when I was hungry
- **2** I ate what I really wanted
- **3** I ate consciously
- **4** I stopped when full
- **5** I drank water
- **6** I moved my body
- **7** I listened to the CD
- **8** I did the mirror exercise

IT'S NOT THAT SOME PEOPLE HAVE WILLPOWER AND SOME DON'T. IT'S THAT SOME PEOPLE ARE READY TO CHANGE AND OTHERS ARE NOT.

JAMES GORDON

You are now more than a third of the way through this 90-day programme. You have set yourself apart from the vast 'herd' of people who say they want to change but are unwilling to do anything to make it happen.

While you celebrate your discipline and perseverance (yes, I'm talking to you!), take some time today to review the week just gone and look forward to the week ahead . . .

1. The best things that happened this week were:

2. My biggest challenges this week were:

3. I did these things for the first time:

4. What I learned was:

5. My top three priorities for the week ahead are:

a.

b.

c.

One **Positive Thing**
I Noticed Today . . .

What I'm **Looking Forward To**
Tomorrow . . .

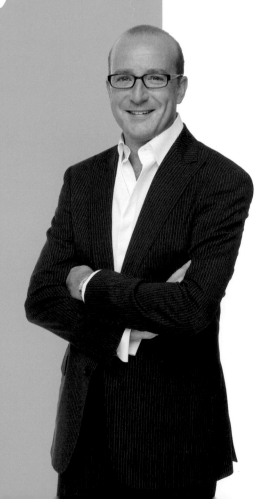

> **IT IS JUST ABOUT IMPOSSIBLE TO SAY GRACE OVER A BINGE.**
>
> VICTORIA MORAN

WEEK 6

EMOTIONAL EATING

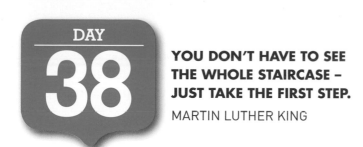

DAY 38

YOU DON'T HAVE TO SEE THE WHOLE STAIRCASE – JUST TAKE THE FIRST STEP.
MARTIN LUTHER KING

FEELING YOUR FEELINGS

What are you feeling right now?

Instead of going to your head for a verbal answer, take ten seconds or so to scan your physical body from your head down to your stomach. Whatever sensations you notice, I want you to just stay with them for at least 10 seconds . . .

Have the sensations begun to change?

Every time you allow yourself to feel the feeling sensations in your body, instead of cutting off from them or trying to cover them over with food or some other mood-altering substance, those feeling sensations will begin to change.

And when you allow your feeling sensations to flow and change, you will ultimately get to claim the reward of feeling sensational!

TODAY'S SUCCESS CHECKLIST

1. ☐ I ate when I was hungry

2. ☐ I ate what I really wanted

3. ☐ I ate consciously

4. ☐ I stopped when full

5. ☐ I drank water

6. ☐ I moved my body

7. ☐ I listened to the CD

8. ☐ I did the mirror exercise

One **Positive Thing** I Noticed Today . . .

What I'm **Looking Forward To** Tomorrow . . .

1️⃣ I ate when I was hungry

2️⃣ I ate what I really wanted

3️⃣ I ate consciously

4️⃣ I stopped when full

5️⃣ I drank water

6️⃣ I moved my body

7️⃣ I listened to the CD

8️⃣ I did the mirror exercise

One **Positive Thing**
I Noticed Today . . .

What I'm **Looking Forward To**
Tomorrow . . .

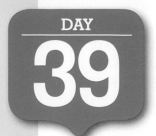

DAY 39

THERE IS NO THINKING WITHOUT FEELING AND NO FEELING WITHOUT THINKING.
KAREN MCCOWN

DEVELOPING YOUR EMOTIONAL INTELLIGENCE

Emotions are messages from your unconscious mind. By taking the time to tune into your body and feel your feelings, you are opening up the channels of communication. Here's a simple process from my book Instant Confidence! that you can use in order to learn from your emotions:

1 Clarify the emotion you're finding uncomfortable. Don't be distracted by WHY you are feeling it – just focus on the feeling itself. Where in your body do you feel it? Are there certain situations, times, places or people with whom it tends to arise?

2 Next, ask yourself what the feeling is about – what message does it have for you? If you're not sure, it's OK to guess – whatever you guess will inevitably come directly from your intuitive self.

3 Whatever the message, let your unconscious mind know you've received it. If there is any action to be taken, promise yourself you will take it as soon as possible – ideally within the next 24 hours.

4 You'll know you've correctly identified the emotion and its message when the uncomfortable feeling begins to dissolve into the background and your natural, confident sense of ease and wellbeing returns to the fore.

DAY 40

WHAT'S EATING YOU?

The number-one reason people eat when they're not hungry is to fill an emotional hole. If you're not used to tuning into your body and feeling your feelings, it can be easy to confuse emotional hunger for its physical equivalent.

Here are the two key things to pay attention to:

1 Emotional hunger is sudden and urgent; physical hunger is gradual and patient.

2 Emotional hunger cannot be satisfied with food; physical hunger can.

If you find yourself eating and eating without getting full, you probably don't need more food – you need love.

Throughout the day today, send yourself love at least once an hour and notice the positive difference it makes!

> **THERE AREN'T ENOUGH COOKIES IN THE WORLD TO MAKE YOU FEEL LOVED AND WHOLE.**
> MICHAEL NEILL

TODAY'S SUCCESS CHECKLIST

- [1] I ate when I was hungry
- [2] I ate what I really wanted
- [3] I ate consciously
- [4] I stopped when full
- [5] I drank water
- [6] I moved my body
- [7] I listened to the CD
- [8] I did the mirror exercise

One **Positive Thing** I Noticed Today . . .

What I'm **Looking Forward To** Tomorrow . . .

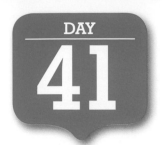

THE PLATINUM RULE

TOO OFTEN WE UNDERESTIMATE THE POWER OF A TOUCH, A SMILE, A KIND WORD, A LISTENING EAR, AN HONEST COMPLIMENT OR THE SMALLEST ACT OF CARING, ALL OF WHICH HAVE THE POTENTIAL TO TURN A LIFE AROUND.

LEO BUSCAGLIA

We are always willing to take more abuse from ourselves than we would ever accept from anyone else. I believe the most important rule when it comes to how you treat yourself is this:

Do unto yourself as you would have others do unto you.

If you want to be treated better, begin by treating yourself better. Do this exercise at least five times today:

1 Ask yourself: 'How can I take better care of myself right now?'

2 Do it!

TODAY'S SUCCESS CHECKLIST

1 I ate when I was hungry

2 I ate what I really wanted

3 I ate consciously

4 I stopped when full

5 I drank water

6 I moved my body

7 I listened to the CD

8 I did the mirror exercise

One **Positive Thing** I Noticed Today . . .

....

....

....

What I'm **Looking Forward To** Tomorrow . . .

....

....

....

DAY 42

CAUGHT IN THE ACT

I MUST LEARN TO LOVE THE FOOL IN ME, THE ONE WHO FEELS TOO MUCH, TALKS TOO MUCH, TAKES TOO MANY CHANCES, WINS SOMETIMES AND LOSES OFTEN, LACKS SELF-CONTROL, LOVES AND HATES, HURTS AND GETS HURT, PROMISES AND BREAKS PROMISES, LAUGHS AND CRIES.

THEODORE ISAAC RUBIN

Here is an excellent exercise from **Change Your Life in 7 Days** that will transform your relationship with your 'inner critic':

1 Stop for a moment and talk to yourself in your critical voice, saying all those nasty things in that unpleasant tone.

2 Now, notice where you make that voice. Does it seem to be coming from inside your head or outside? Is it at the front, the sides or the back?

3 Extend your arm and stick out your thumb.

4 Wherever the critical voice was, move it down your arm to the tip of your thumb, so it's now speaking to you from there.

5 Next slow it down and change the tone of it. Make it sound sexy, or speed it up so it sounds like Mickey Mouse.

TODAY'S SUCCESS CHECKLIST

1 I ate when I was hungry

2 I ate what I really wanted

3 I ate consciously

4 I stopped when full

5 I drank water

6 I moved my body

7 I listened to the CD

8 I did the mirror exercise

One **Positive Thing** I Noticed Today . . .

What I'm **Looking Forward To** Tomorrow . . .

195

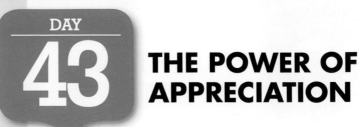
THE POWER OF APPRECIATION

Here are some wonderful questions for you to ask and answer throughout the day today:

1 What's right with my life?

2 What's working?

3 Who do I love and who loves me?

4 What am I most grateful for in my life?

The real value in this exercise is not just the good feelings you will experience in your body but also the changes it will make in your life. By taking the time to deliberately appreciate what you already like and love, you invoke the law of increase:

You get more of what you focus on!

> **THE DEEPEST PRINCIPAL IN HUMAN NATURE IS THE CRAVING TO BE APPRECIATED.**
> WILLIAM JAMES

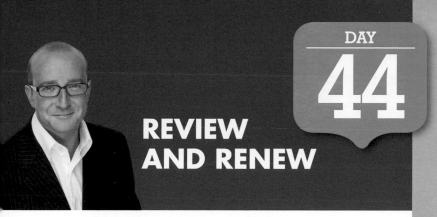

REVIEW AND RENEW

TODAY'S SUCCESS CHECKLIST

- [ ] **1** I ate when I was hungry
- [ ] **2** I ate what I really wanted
- [ ] **3** I ate consciously
- [ ] **4** I stopped when full
- [ ] **5** I drank water
- [ ] **6** I moved my body
- [ ] **7** I listened to the CD
- [ ] **8** I did the mirror exercise

SOMETIMES IT'S THE SMALLEST DECISIONS THAT CAN CHANGE YOUR LIFE FOR EVER.

KERI RUSSELL

So, how are you feeling right now? Today is an excellent day to reconnect with a supportive friend as you ask and answer the following questions . . .

1. The best things that happened this week were:

....

2. My biggest challenges this week were:

....

3. I did these things for the first time:

....

4. What I learned was:

....

5. My top three priorities for the week ahead are:

a. ....

b. ....

c. ....

One **Positive Thing** I Noticed Today . . .

....

....

What I'm **Looking Forward To** Tomorrow . . .

....

....

....

YOUR THIRD CHECK-IN . . .

Can you believe it? You're already halfway through! If you're like most people, you're probably feeling one of three ways:

- **Excited about your changing body shape and the additional changes that are happening in your life.**
- **Cautiously optimistic – the physical changes haven't been as dramatic as you'd hoped yet, but you can tell that things are different to the way they were before.**
- **Stuck, frustrated and contemplating giving up. You haven't lost much weight, and you're beginning to question me, yourself and the system.**

Whichever way you're feeling right now, the most important thing is to keep going. Now that you have a better understanding of what it's like to eat in this new way, you are able to recommit to the programme (and yourself!) at a whole new level. Fill in your new commitment below:

'I, _____, commit to finishing this bloody programme and giving myself a real chance to succeed no matter how I feel about it!'

TODAY I WEIGH

YVONNE MEANEY

LOST

6½

STONE

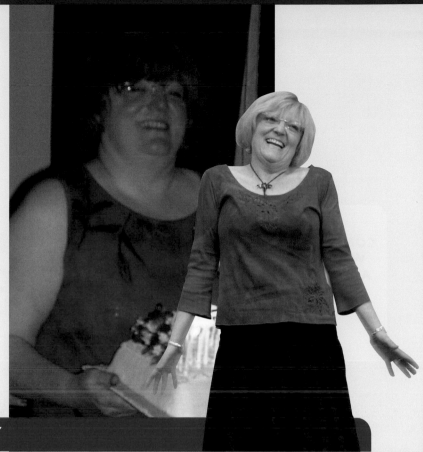

YVONNE'S STORY

I had dieted often over the years. I'd lose weight, then put it all back on, plus extra. I got heavier and heavier, until I was over 16 stone, depressed, unhappy and convinced I'd be fat for life.

My husband lost weight using Paul's book and CD, and nagged me to try it. I started following the four golden rules. When I began to lose weight, I realized there was something to this system, so I read Paul's book. The section on exercise encouraged me to start walking. I started with 2,000 extra steps a day and found I enjoyed it. I got quicker and went further and ended up running. It seemed the more I did, the lighter I became, the easier it got and the more I did . . .

Ten months later I had lost 6 1/2 stone and since then I haven't looked back. Running is now part of my life and I've taken part in many races, including marathons. Using this system has been life-changing. It was never a struggle, I never binged or felt miserable. It has given me complete freedom around food. I've gone from Couch Potato to Marathon Runner, and the weight has gone for good.

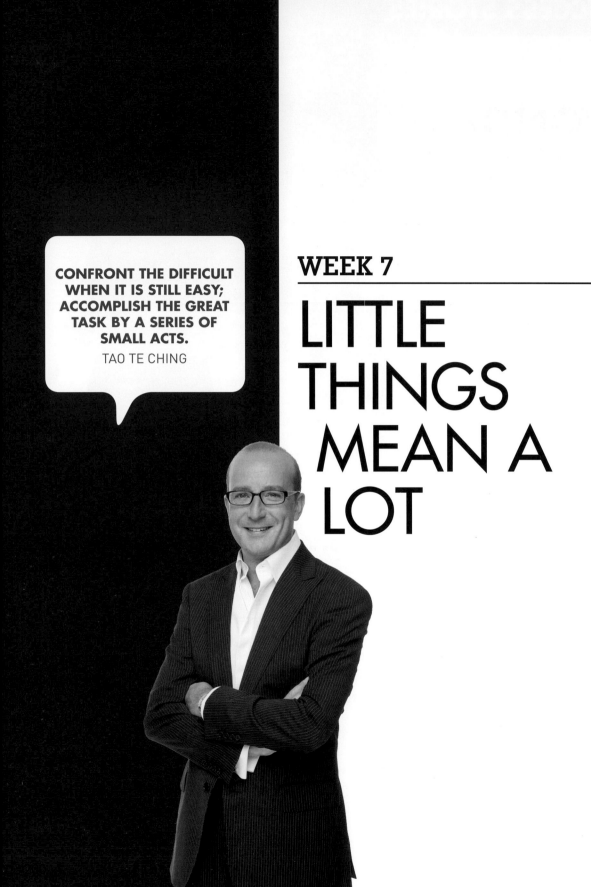

> CONFRONT THE DIFFICULT
> WHEN IT IS STILL EASY;
> ACCOMPLISH THE GREAT
> TASK BY A SERIES OF
> SMALL ACTS.
>
> TAO TE CHING

WEEK 7

LITTLE THINGS MEAN A LOT

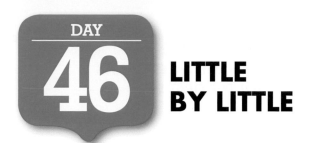

DAY 46

LITTLE BY LITTLE

CONTINUAL IMPROVEMENT IS AN UNENDING JOURNEY.

LLOYD DOBENS

Do little things really mean a lot? Highly successful Japanese corporations often put their achievements down to the practice of kaizen – a philosophy of continual improvement where small daily actions lead to major lasting changes. To practise kaizen in your own life, consider the words of John Wooden, one of the most successful basketball coaches in history:

'When you improve a little each day, eventually big things occur. When you improve conditioning a little each day, eventually you have a big improvement in conditioning. Not tomorrow, not the next day, but eventually a big gain is made. Don't look for the big, quick improvement. Seek the small improvement, one day at a time. That's the only way it happens – and when it happens, it lasts.'

What are the three smallest changes you could implement this week that might make the biggest difference to your ability to follow through with this programme? Write them down.

Now do them!

TODAY'S SUCCESS CHECKLIST

1. I ate when I was hungry

2. I ate what I really wanted

3. I ate consciously

4. I stopped when full

5. I drank water

6. I moved my body

7. I listened to the CD

8. I did the mirror exercise

One **Positive Thing** I Noticed Today . . .

What I'm **Looking Forward To** Tomorrow . . .

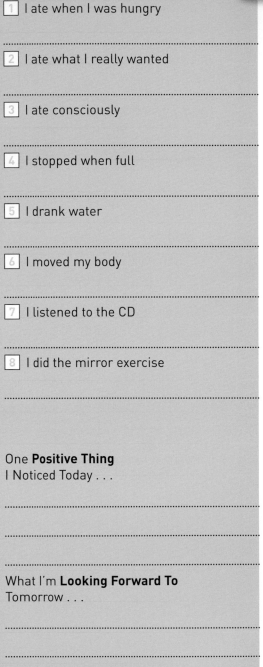

TODAY'S SUCCESS CHECKLIST

1 I ate when I was hungry

2 I ate what I really wanted

3 I ate consciously

4 I stopped when full

5 I drank water

6 I moved my body

7 I listened to the CD

8 I did the mirror exercise

One **Positive Thing**
I Noticed Today . . .

What I'm **Looking Forward To**
Tomorrow . . .

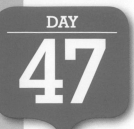

DAY
47

A JOURNEY OF A THOUSAND MILES BEGINS WITH THE FIRST STEP.
LAO TZU

STEP BY STEP

Dr James Hill discovered there was a difference of only 1,500 to 2,000 steps taken a day between people who were overweight and those who maintained a healthy weight. That may sound like a lot, but it's only about four city blocks. Get creative with at least ten ways you can 'step up' your physical movement today. Here are a couple of suggestions to get you started . . .

Taking the steps instead of the elevator.
Walking to work.

I can move more today by:

1

2

3

4

5

6

7

8

9

10

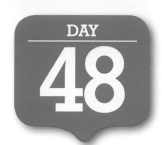

BIT BY BIT

IF YOU JUST KEEP MOVING, SOONER OR LATER THE FINISH LINE WILL SHOW UP.

STU MITTLEMAN

Stu Mittleman is the world record holder for the 1,000-mile endurance run and a physical mastery 'guru'. In an interview I once read, a reporter asked Mittleman how he had geared up mentally for running the equivalent of nearly 40 continuous marathons. Mittleman replied:

'I never ran 1,000 miles – I can't even conceive of running 1,000 miles. All I did was run one mile a thousand times.'

Do you believe you could lose one pound this week by continuing to eat when you're hungry and stopping when you think you're full?

If so, congratulations – you WILL reach your goal!

TODAY'S SUCCESS CHECKLIST

1 I ate when I was hungry

2 I ate what I really wanted

3 I ate consciously

4 I stopped when full

5 I drank water

6 I moved my body

7 I listened to the CD

8 I did the mirror exercise

One **Positive Thing** I Noticed Today . . .

....

....

What I'm **Looking Forward To** Tomorrow . . .

....

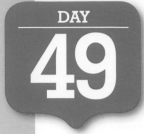
ONE BY ONE

YOU CANNOT CHANGE YOUR DESTINATION OVERNIGHT, BUT YOU CAN CHANGE YOUR DIRECTION OVERNIGHT. JIM ROHN

TODAY'S SUCCESS CHECKLIST

1. ☐ I ate when I was hungry

2. ☐ I ate what I really wanted

3. ☐ I ate consciously

4. ☐ I stopped when full

5. ☐ I drank water

6. ☐ I moved my body

7. ☐ I listened to the CD

8. ☐ I did the mirror exercise

One **Positive Thing**
I Noticed Today . . .

What I'm **Looking Forward To**
Tomorrow . . .

There is a part of your brain called the amygdala whose job is to keep you safe by preventing you from making major changes in your life. Any time it senses you're going to upset the status quo, it releases stress hormones into your body to 'encourage' you to give up and go back to 'the way things always have been'.

Taking one small action a day outsmarts the amygdala by sneaking past its radar. Yet the cumulative effects of these single daily actions will be nothing short of life-changing. When you are used to doing one thing, two things is easy. When you are used to doing fifty, fifty-one is just as simple.

What is one small daily action you could begin taking to make changes in the important areas of your life?

Here are some examples to get you started . . .

To manage stress, I will take one deep breath a day
To save money, I will put one penny into a jar
To have more time, I will get up one minute earlier than usual

Now it's your turn . . .

To move my body more, I will: _____

To enjoy my life more, I will: _____

To be kinder to myself, I will: _____

PICTURE BY PICTURE

ALL GREAT THINGS HAVE SMALL BEGINNINGS.

PETER SENGE

Here is a simple way to create a powerful image of yourself being exactly the way you want to be:

1 Imagine a slightly slimmer you sitting or standing in front of you.

2 Now, I'd like you to imagine stepping into that slimmer you. See through their eyes, hear through their ears and feel the feelings of your slimmer, more radiant self. And notice that right in front of you is an even slimmer you – sitting or standing a little bit taller, a look of slightly more self-belief behind the eyes, emanating a little bit of extra charisma.

3 Step into this slimmer, more radiant self, and notice that in front of you is an even slimmer self – more self-assured and radiating even more inner beauty.

4 Repeat step three, stepping into slimmer and slimmer versions of yourself until you are looking through the eyes of your naturally slim and radiant self. Be sure to notice how you are using your body – how you are breathing, the expression on your face and the light in your eyes.

Enjoy!

TODAY'S SUCCESS CHECKLIST

1 I ate when I was hungry

2 I ate what I really wanted

3 I ate consciously

4 I stopped when full

5 I drank water

6 I moved my body

7 I listened to the CD

8 I did the mirror exercise

One **Positive Thing** I Noticed Today . . .

What I'm **Looking Forward To** Tomorrow . . .

- [1] I ate when I was hungry
- [2] I ate what I really wanted
- [3] I ate consciously
- [4] I stopped when full
- [5] I drank water
- [6] I moved my body
- [7] I listened to the CD
- [8] I did the mirror exercise

One **Positive Thing**
I Noticed Today . . .

What I'm **Looking Forward To**
Tomorrow . . .

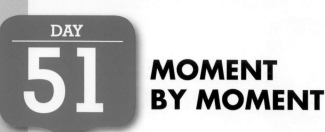

DAY 51
MOMENT BY MOMENT

Just for today, collect moments. Perhaps you will see a child hugging its mother and you will experience a moment of unconditional love. Later, a friend will call and you'll have a moment of excitement as you learn something new about a mutual acquaintance. Then you'll be out for a walk and the sun will catch your eye in a way that evokes a moment of timelessness.

Normally we walk right by these moments in our lives, distracted by the pursuit of 'more important' things like cooking dinner for the family, finishing the laundry or watching our favourite soap opera.

Today, collect as many of them as you can . . .

> **SUCCESS IS HOW YOU COLLECT YOUR MINUTES . . . IF YOU DON'T HAVE ALL OF THOSE ZILLIONS OF TINY SUCCESSES, THE BIG ONES DON'T MEAN ANYTHING.**
>
> NORMAN LEAR

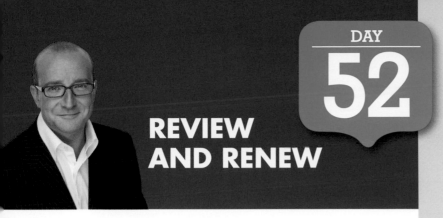

52

REVIEW AND RENEW

TO GOD, THERE IS NOTHING SMALL.

MOTHER TERESA

Day by day and week by week, you are becoming the person you have dreamt about for all these years. Today, take time out to review, renew and celebrate how far you've already come . . .

1. The best things that happened this week were:

....

2. My biggest challenges this week were:

....

3. I did these things for the first time:

....

4. What I learned was:

....

5. My top three priorities for the week ahead are:

a. ....

b. ....

c. ....

TODAY'S SUCCESS CHECKLIST

- ☐ 1 I ate when I was hungry
- ☐ 2 I ate what I really wanted
- ☐ 3 I ate consciously
- ☐ 4 I stopped when full
- ☐ 5 I drank water
- ☐ 6 I moved my body
- ☐ 7 I listened to the CD
- ☐ 8 I did the mirror exercise

One **Positive Thing**
I Noticed Today . . .

....

....

What I'm **Looking Forward To**
Tomorrow . . .

....

....

....

WEEK 8

EATING CONSCIOUSLY

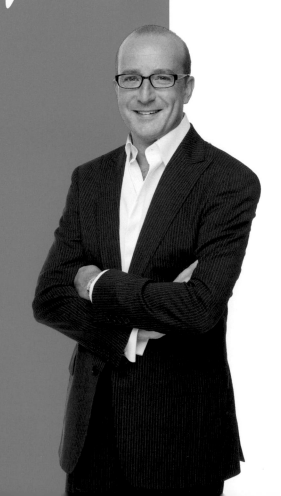

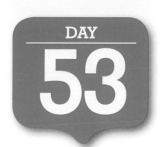

DAY 53

THE BREEZE FROM THE REFRIGERATOR DOOR

MINDFULNESS CAN BE SUMMED UP IN TWO WORDS: PAY ATTENTION. ONCE YOU NOTICE WHAT YOU'RE DOING, YOU HAVE THE POWER TO CHANGE IT.

MICHELLE BURFORD

Here's a simple way to become more mindful and present in any moment:

1 Notice three things you can see.

2 Notice three things you can hear.

3 Notice three things you can feel.

Practise this throughout the day today, particularly when you are preparing your meals and sitting down to eat.

When you become really present, you may even notice the breeze as you close the refrigerator door!

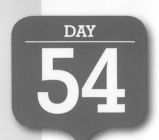

TODAY'S SUCCESS CHECKLIST

1. ☐ I ate when I was hungry

2. ☐ I ate what I really wanted

3. ☐ I ate consciously

4. ☐ I stopped when full

5. ☐ I drank water

6. ☐ I moved my body

7. ☐ I listened to the CD

8. ☐ I did the mirror exercise

One **Positive Thing**
I Noticed Today . . .

....

....

....

What I'm **Looking Forward To**
Tomorrow . . .

....

....

....

SMELL YOURSELF SLIM

NOTHING IS MORE MEMORABLE THAN A SMELL. ONE SCENT CAN BE UNEXPECTED, MOMENTARY AND FLEETING, YET CONJURE UP A CHILDHOOD SUMMER BESIDE A LAKE IN THE MOUNTAINS; ANOTHER, A MOONLIT BEACH; A THIRD, A FAMILY DINNER OF POT ROAST AND SWEET POTATOES DURING A MYRTLE-MAD AUGUST IN A MIDWESTERN TOWN.

DIANE ACKERMAN

According to Dr Richard Bandler, taking a few moments to smell each bite of food before putting it in your mouth alerts your brain to what you are about to eat. Your brain then triggers the correct digestive enzymes to be released into both your saliva and your stomach, and whatever you are eating will be digested quickly and efficiently.

Today, take the time to smell each bite of food before you eat it. You'll find it will not only enhance your ability to enjoy each mouthful, you'll feel better afterwards as well.

What do you do if you don't like the smell?

Don't eat it!

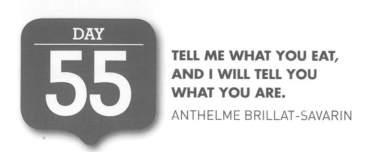

TELL ME WHAT YOU EAT, AND I WILL TELL YOU WHAT YOU ARE.

ANTHELME BRILLAT-SAVARIN

WRITE IT DOWN!

You've already learned in keeping this journal that there is an incredible value in writing down what you are doing as you are doing it, and in taking the time to review what you have done and to learn from it.

Today, increase your mindfulness of what you put into your body by writing EVERYTHING down, from the sugar-free breath mint to the evening cup of tea. This is not to make yourself feel guilty about what you are eating – remember, there is no such thing as a forbidden food. It is simply to assist you in becoming more and more aware . . .

Morning:

Afternoon:

Early Evening:

Late Evening:

TODAY'S SUCCESS CHECKLIST

1. I ate when I was hungry

2. I ate what I really wanted

3. I ate consciously

4. I stopped when full

5. I drank water

6. I moved my body

7. I listened to the CD

8. I did the mirror exercise

One **Positive Thing**
I Noticed Today . . .

What I'm **Looking Forward To**
Tomorrow . . .

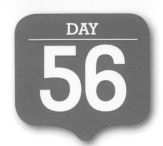

SOCIAL MINDFULNESS

IT COMES AS A GREAT SHOCK TO PEOPLE THAT THEY CAN SOCIALIZE WITHOUT SHOVING FOOD IN THEIR MOUTHS.

DAVE BARRY

One of the first questions I've learned to ask people who are finding it difficult to lose weight is, 'Are you eating consciously?'

Although they always say yes, it often turns out that they habitually eat in social gatherings, chatting away throughout the meal. While it's not impossible to stay conscious and mindful of what you are eating while you are also engaged in conversation, it is bloody difficult.

Just for today, experiment with eating when you eat and socializing when you socialize – you may be surprised at the difference it makes!

TODAY'S SUCCESS CHECKLIST

1 I ate when I was hungry

2 I ate what I really wanted

3 I ate consciously

4 I stopped when full

5 I drank water

6 I moved my body

7 I listened to the CD

8 I did the mirror exercise

One **Positive Thing** I Noticed Today . . .

What I'm **Looking Forward To** Tomorrow . . .

BREAK WITH ROUTINE

FORTUNE AND LOVE BEFRIEND THE BOLD.

OVID

One excellent way to become more conscious of your eating is to change your eating routines. Your conscious mind loves it when you do something the same way every time because it leaves it free to pay attention to something else.

But when it comes to eating, we want to keep our minds front and centre, present and accounted for. What are some of your habitual eating routines?

Do you always eat at a certain time, or in a certain place in the kitchen or sitting room? Do you use the same plates, glasses and cutlery?

Today, change at least one thing from your eating routine. This could be as simple as moving your couch or TV into a slightly different position, or shifting the furniture in your kitchen around. If you're doing it right, it should feel a little bit odd, and maybe even slightly uncomfortable.

As soon as you start getting used to the new way, it's time to break with routine once again!

TODAY'S SUCCESS CHECKLIST

- [1] I ate when I was hungry
- [2] I ate what I really wanted
- [3] I ate consciously
- [4] I stopped when full
- [5] I drank water
- [6] I moved my body
- [7] I listened to the CD
- [8] I did the mirror exercise

One **Positive Thing** I Noticed Today . . .

What I'm **Looking Forward To** Tomorrow . . .

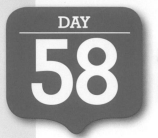

DAY 58

OVERCOMING BOREDOM

1. I ate when I was hungry

2. I ate what I really wanted

3. I ate consciously

4. I stopped when full

5. I drank water

6. I moved my body

7. I listened to the CD

8. I did the mirror exercise

One **Positive Thing**
I Noticed Today . . .

What I'm **Looking Forward To**
Tomorrow . . .

LIFE IS NO BRIEF CANDLE TO ME. IT IS A SORT OF SPLENDID TORCH WHICH I HAVE GOT A HOLD OF FOR THE MOMENT, AND I WANT TO MAKE IT BURN AS BRIGHTLY AS POSSIBLE BEFORE HANDING IT ONTO FUTURE GENERATIONS.

GEORGE BERNARD SHAW

I have a friend whose young daughter is continually bored. When she can no longer stand to hear her daughter complain, she fixes her a snack.

Allow me to let you in on a little secret:

The cure for boredom is activity, not food.

If you find yourself feeling bored today, in search of something to do, move your body. Go for a walk. Dance. Your mind will thank you and your body will be beside itself with joy!

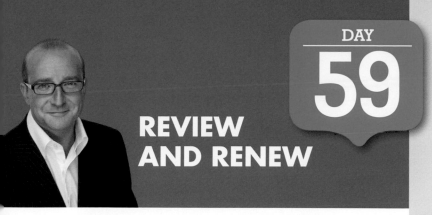

REVIEW AND RENEW

TODAY'S SUCCESS CHECKLIST

- [1] I ate when I was hungry
- [2] I ate what I really wanted
- [3] I ate consciously
- [4] I stopped when full
- [5] I drank water
- [6] I moved my body
- [7] I listened to the CD
- [8] I did the mirror exercise

REFLECT UPON YOUR PRESENT BLESSINGS, OF WHICH EVERY MAN HAS MANY; NOT UPON YOUR PAST MISFORTUNES, OF WHICH ALL MEN HAVE SOME.

CHARLES DICKENS

Did you enjoy your week of eating mindfully? It doesn't have to end today – as you move into the final month of our time together, mindfulness can be a powerful ally as you continue to reprogram your mind and body to be naturally thin. Take some time today to ask and answer these questions . . .

1. The best things that happened this week were:

....

2. My biggest challenges this week were:

....

3. I did these things for the first time:

....

4. What I learned was:

....

5. My top three priorities for the week ahead are:

a.
....

b.
....

c.
....

One **Positive Thing**
I Noticed Today . . .

....

....

What I'm **Looking Forward To**
Tomorrow . . .

....

....

....

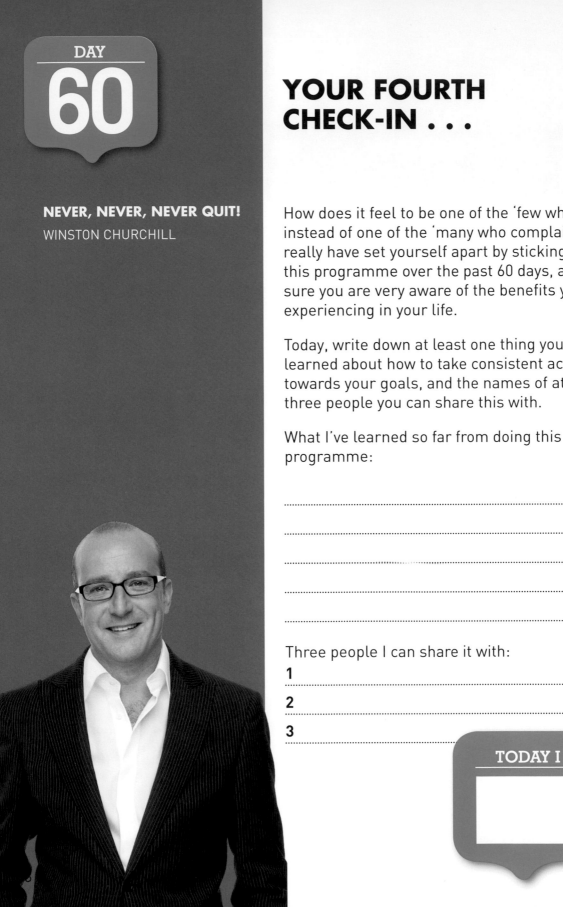

DAY
60

NEVER, NEVER, NEVER QUIT!
WINSTON CHURCHILL

YOUR FOURTH CHECK-IN . . .

How does it feel to be one of the 'few who do' instead of one of the 'many who complain'? You really have set yourself apart by sticking with this programme over the past 60 days, and I'm sure you are very aware of the benefits you are experiencing in your life.

Today, write down at least one thing you've learned about how to take consistent action towards your goals, and the names of at least three people you can share this with.

What I've learned so far from doing this programme:

....

....

....

....

....

Three people I can share it with:

1 ....

2 ....

3 ....

TODAY I WEIGH

GILLIAN TODHUNTER

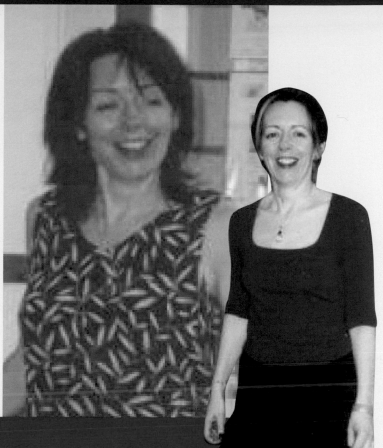

LOST
2½
STONE

GILLIAN'S STORY

I was 11 stone, 3 pounds: overweight, lethargic, lacking in self-esteem and with poor concentration. It was time for action. I went to Weight Watchers. I reached my target weight, but all I could think about was food. After a while I piled back on all the weight I'd lost and more, until I reached my heaviest ever: over 12 stone.

I bought Paul McKenna's Easy Weight-Loss CDs, and listened to them in the comfort of our home. Very soon, I was filled with positive willpower. I began to change my attitude towards food and my body. I learned how to listen to and understand my own body's signals. The weight began to disappear, quickly and easily. I reached my target weight of 10 stone – and what's more, I've stayed there. Five years on and I still weigh 10 stone, and food and eating no longer occupy every thought. My old eating habits have been replaced. I am now vegetarian, and my new-found confidence has seen me change my job and the way I exercise. This new confidence, which has come from not having to worry about my body size, has helped me become a person with a positive outlook on life.

> **ANGELS FLY BECAUSE THEY TAKE THEMSELVES LIGHTLY.**
> G.K. CHESTERTON

WEEK 9
LIGHTEN UP!

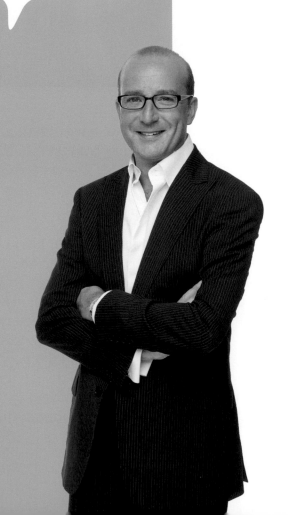

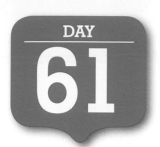

COMING OUT OF THE CLOSET

WHEN I BUY COOKIES I EAT JUST FOUR AND THROW THE REST AWAY. BUT FIRST I SPRAY THEM WITH INSECT REPELLENT SO I WON'T DIG THEM OUT OF THE GARBAGE LATER. BE CAREFUL, THOUGH, BECAUSE THAT INSECT REPELLENT REALLY DOESN'T TASTE THAT BAD.

JANETTE BARBER

What's the craziest thing you've ever done to hide your obsession with food?

Whatever the answer, one of the most powerful things you can do is to go public with it. While I don't normally find myself agreeing with Sigmund Freud, he said one thing I totally concur with:

Our secrets make us sick.

Today, 'come out of the closet' about something you've been keeping secret. Make sure you do so with a good friend, and don't be surprised if they try to top you with a 'secret story' of their own!

TODAY'S SUCCESS CHECKLIST

1. ☐ I ate when I was hungry

2. ☐ I ate what I really wanted

3. ☐ I ate consciously

4. ☐ I stopped when full

5. ☐ I drank water

6. ☐ I moved my body

7. ☐ I listened to the CD

8. ☐ I did the mirror exercise

One **Positive Thing** I Noticed Today . . .

What I'm **Looking Forward To** Tomorrow . . .

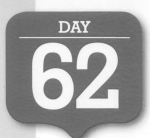
TODAY'S SUCCESS CHECKLIST

1. ☐ I ate when I was hungry

2. ☐ I ate what I really wanted

3. ☐ I ate consciously

4. ☐ I stopped when full

5. ☐ I drank water

6. ☐ I moved my body

7. ☐ I listened to the CD

8. ☐ I did the mirror exercise

One **Positive Thing**
I Noticed Today . . .

What I'm **Looking Forward To**
Tomorrow . . .

THE BEST MEDICINE

LAUGHTER HAS NO LANGUAGE, KNOWS NO BOUNDARIES, DOES NOT DISCRIMINATE BETWEEN CASTE, CREED AND COLOUR. IT IS A POWERFUL EMOTION AND HAS ALL THE INGREDIENTS FOR UNITING THE ENTIRE WORLD.

DR MADAN KATARIA

According to studies, children laugh up to 400 times a day and adults just 15 times a day. Which to me is proof that there's just too much seriousness in the world!

Madan Kataria MD is known as 'the laughter doctor'. He has founded laughter groups all over the world where people meet to practise 'yogic laughing' for about 15 minutes every day. Yogic laughing is a technique where people are encouraged to laugh for no reason. The reason it is so powerful is that when we pretend to laugh or act happy, our bodies cannot tell the difference between real and pretend and release all the happy positive health chemicals inside us that make us feel good.

So today, whenever it's appropriate (and at least once when it's not!), laugh out loud for as long as you can and kick-start the happy chemicals in your body!

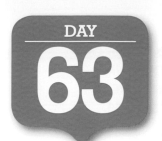

THE SECOND DAY OF A DIET IS ALWAYS EASIER THAN THE FIRST. BY THE SECOND DAY, YOU'RE OFF IT.

JACKIE GLEASON

NAME THE GAME

Every day, we are bombarded with messages telling us not only that we aren't good enough as we are, but that if we will only try this diet or this eating plan, everything will be all right. Today, make note of the many different ways you are invited by television, advertising, shops, newspapers and magazines to ignore what your body wants and eat what the 'experts' tell you is good for you instead.

Here are some to get you started . . .

1. Fat-free
2. No sugar added
3. Free inside –
    10 tips to lose those last 10 pounds!
4. As recommended by . . .

And here's space for your own . . .

5

6

7

8

9

10

TODAY'S SUCCESS CHECKLIST

1. I ate when I was hungry

2. I ate what I really wanted

3. I ate consciously

4. I stopped when full

5. I drank water

6. I moved my body

7. I listened to the CD

8. I did the mirror exercise

One **Positive Thing**
I Noticed Today . . .

What I'm **Looking Forward To**
Tomorrow . . .

1. ☐ I ate when I was hungry

2. ☐ I ate what I really wanted

3. ☐ I ate consciously

4. ☐ I stopped when full

5. ☐ I drank water

6. ☐ I moved my body

7. ☐ I listened to the CD

8. ☐ I did the mirror exercise

One **Positive Thing**
I Noticed Today . . .

What I'm **Looking Forward To**
Tomorrow . . .

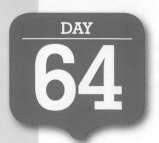

DAY 64

THERE ARE TWO KINDS OF LIGHT – THE GLOW THAT ILLUMINATES AND THE GLARE THAT OBSCURES.

JAMES THURBER

A BODY OF LIGHT

An American research study showed that visualizing your body filled with light has a powerful positive effect upon your health and feelings of wellbeing. Here's a simple exercise you can use to connect with that light. As your body grows lighter and lighter, imagine it becoming more and more beautiful . . .

1 Imagine you are preparing your body to bring in more light. What can you do to make your body comfortable and your energy as attractive as possible?

2 Take a deep breath and invite light into your body. Imagine it filling your spine and radiating throughout your entire body, until every cell is alive and filled with light.

3 Extend the light out beyond the limits of your physical body. Imagine it radiating out to fill the room, or gently surrounding you like a cocoon. Keep playing with it until it feels just right to you.

4 Now imagine you are sending this light to the person or situation that needs it most. Don't worry about running out – the more you share the light, the more your own is replenished.

This is an excellent way to recharge yourself whenever you need a boost of mental, physical or spiritual energy. Use it as often as you like!

DAY 65 — PRONOIA IN ACTION

YOU SHOULD VIEW THE WORLD AS A CONSPIRACY RUN BY A VERY CLOSELY KNIT GROUP OF NEARLY OMNIPOTENT PEOPLE, AND YOU SHOULD THINK OF THOSE PEOPLE AS YOURSELF AND YOUR FRIENDS.

ROBERT ANTON WILSON

I believe there should be a new category of mental health called 'pronoia' – the belief that everything and everyone is conspiring to do you good! Here's a simple way to put pronoia into action . . .

Just for today, live as if there is a positive benefit in every one of life's events. Jot down something that happened today and find (or make up!) the positive benefit . . .

What happened: *I ate about five more biscuits than I intended.*

This is good because: *It shows how much I've changed – in the past I would have eaten the whole box!*

What happened:

This is good because:

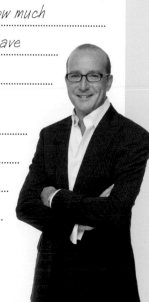

223

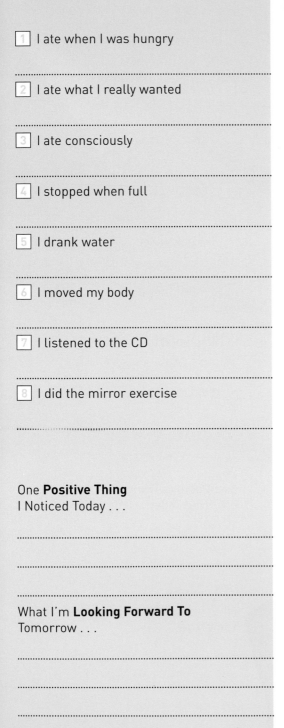

- ☐ 1 I ate when I was hungry
- ☐ 2 I ate what I really wanted
- ☐ 3 I ate consciously
- ☐ 4 I stopped when full
- ☐ 5 I drank water
- ☐ 6 I moved my body
- ☐ 7 I listened to the CD
- ☐ 8 I did the mirror exercise

One **Positive Thing**
I Noticed Today . . .

What I'm **Looking Forward To**
Tomorrow . . .

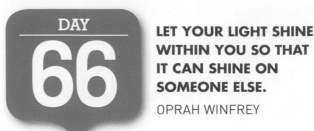

DAY 66

LET YOUR LIGHT SHINE WITHIN YOU SO THAT IT CAN SHINE ON SOMEONE ELSE.
OPRAH WINFREY

THE LIGHT OF THE WORLD

One of my favourite quotes in the world comes from Marianne Williamson, author of **A Return to Love**:

Our deepest fear is not that we are inadequate. Our deepest fear is that we are powerful beyond measure. It is our light, not our darkness, that most frightens us. We ask ourselves, Who am I to be brilliant, gorgeous, talented, fabulous? Actually, who are you not to be?

You are a child of God. Your playing small does not serve the world. There is nothing enlightened about shrinking so that other people won't feel insecure around you.

We are all meant to shine, as children do. We were born to make manifest the glory of God that is within us. It is not just in some of us; it is in everyone.

And as we let our own light shine, we unconsciously give other people permission to do the same. As we are liberated from our own fear, our presence automatically liberates others.

How can you let your own light shine out into the world today? Whose life can you touch with your presence? Just for today, allow your full magnificence to shine forth!

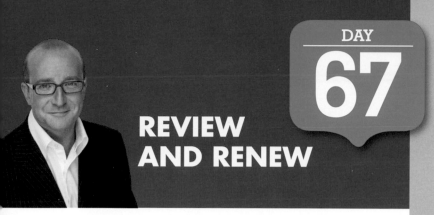

REVIEW AND RENEW

TODAY'S SUCCESS CHECKLIST

IN THE RIGHT LIGHT, AT THE RIGHT TIME, EVERYTHING IS EXTRAORDINARY.

AARON ROSE

By now, you have probably lightened up in more ways than one. As you take the time to review and renew this week, let yourself do so with a light touch and an even lighter heart. Why not invite a friend to join you and share what you've learned?

1. The best things that happened this week were:

....

2. My biggest challenges this week were:

....

3. I did these things for the first time:

....

4. What I learned was:

....

5. My top three priorities for the week ahead are:

a. ....

b. ....

c. ....

- [1] I ate when I was hungry

- [2] I ate what I really wanted

- [3] I ate consciously

- [4] I stopped when full

- [5] I drank water

- [6] I moved my body

- [7] I listened to the CD

- [8] I did the mirror exercise

One **Positive Thing** I Noticed Today . . .

....

....

What I'm **Looking Forward To** Tomorrow . . .

....

....

....

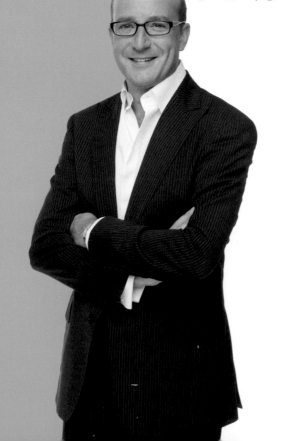

> **THE GREATEST GIFT IS NOT BEING AFRAID TO QUESTION.**
> RUBY DEE

THE WEIGHT-LOSS CLINIC – YOUR QUESTIONS ANSWERED

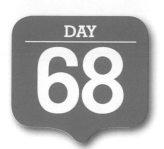

Q: Do I have to eat like this for the rest of my life?

That's a bit like asking if you have to enjoy great sex with the person of your dreams for the rest of your life! Which bits of the system would you like to change?

- **Would you like to stop eating when you're hungry?**
- **Would you like to stop eating the foods you love and want to eat?**
- **Would you like to stop enjoying your food as you eat it?**
- **Would you like to begin making yourself sick from overeating?**

Remember, there's nothing in my system designed to punish you or make you wrong – just a recognition that when you are willing to trust your body and stay conscious, your body will reward you with more energy, more aliveness and less wobble.

TODAY'S SUCCESS CHECKLIST

1. I ate when I was hungry

2. I ate what I really wanted

3. I ate consciously

4. I stopped when full

5. I drank water

6. I moved my body

7. I listened to the CD

8. I did the mirror exercise

One **Positive Thing** I Noticed Today . . .

What I'm **Looking Forward To** Tomorrow . . .

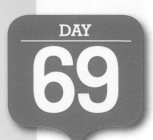
TODAY'S SUCCESS CHECKLIST

1 I ate when I was hungry

2 I ate what I really wanted

3 I ate consciously

4 I stopped when full

5 I drank water

6 I moved my body

7 I listened to the CD

8 I did the mirror exercise

One **Positive Thing**
I Noticed Today . . .

What I'm **Looking Forward To**
Tomorrow . . .

Q: It worked great for the first month, but now it's stopped working. Can I come back to it again after I eat low-fat for a few months?

OK, let's start from the beginning . . .

1 Diets are bad for you. They have been proven to lead to significant weight gain over time, they damage your metabolism and sometimes your health, and they reinforce the myth that someone can know more about what your body needs than you do.

2 I have yet to meet anyone who says, 'The system stopped working', who doesn't mean, 'I stopped using the system'. If you are eating when you are hungry, eating what you really want, enjoying each mouthful and stopping when you think you're full, YOU WILL LOSE WEIGHT or maintain a healthy weight if you're already there.

3 The most common problem I've seen is that after a time, people speed up and begin to go into unconscious eating again. While it's certainly possible to eat quickly and maintain a healthy weight, particularly once your metabolism resets itself, in the meantime, slow your eating down until you are once again completely conscious of each and every mouthful!

DAY 70

Q: Can I 'cheat' and still lose weight?

No, you can't 'cheat' and still lose weight – but not for the reason you think. You can't 'cheat' because there are no foods you can cheat with. Nothing is forbidden – nothing.

Almost all diets agree that there are 'good' foods, 'bad' foods and 'neutral' foods. And, surprisingly perhaps, I agree with them. 'Good' foods are the ones you eat because they taste good, 'bad' foods are the ones you try to convince yourself to eat because they're supposed to be good for you, and neutral foods are the ones you don't eat!

TODAY'S SUCCESS CHECKLIST

1 I ate when I was hungry

2 I ate what I really wanted

3 I ate consciously

4 I stopped when full

5 I drank water

6 I moved my body

7 I listened to the CD

8 I did the mirror exercise

One **Positive Thing** I Noticed Today . . .

....

....

....

What I'm **Looking Forward To** Tomorrow . . .

....

....

....

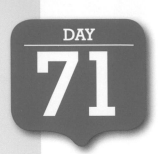

**TODAY'S SUCCESS
CHECKLIST**

☐1 I ate when I was hungry

☐2 I ate what I really wanted

☐3 I ate consciously

☐4 I stopped when full

☐5 I drank water

☐6 I moved my body

☐7 I listened to the CD

☐8 I did the mirror exercise

One **Positive Thing**
I Noticed Today . . .

....

....

....

What I'm **Looking Forward To**
Tomorrow . . .

....

....

....

....

Q: How do I eat at a party? I find it really difficult to keep track of how much I'm eating and usually don't notice I'm full until it's too late!

Many people feel nervous at parties and use food and alcohol to try to control their feelings. But the trick to enjoying a party isn't to eat or drink more; it's to place your attention outside of yourself, on the people around you. This is the exact opposite of what you have been learning in this book – to eat with your attention on your food and your body. This is why when you are learning my system, at least for the first two weeks, I recommend you avoid any situation that you know will throw you back into your old eating habits. Once you've grounded yourself in this new way of eating, you can reintroduce yourself to what used to be difficult situations.

If you still find yourself wanting to change the way you feel at a party, you can always use the tapping exercise (Craving Buster Number 1, on page 118).

Q: I want to eat pasta constantly – is that what my body wants or is it a craving?

The simplest test for a craving is this:

If you can't not eat it, it's a craving.

Fortunately, once you recognize it for what it is, it's the easiest thing in the world to tap it away using Craving Buster Number 1 on page 118.

Ultimately, the way to eliminate a craving for ever is to use Craving Buster Number 2 on page 120 – but be careful! Don't use this unless you're ready to give up eating a particular food forever . . .

TODAY'S SUCCESS CHECKLIST

1 I ate when I was hungry	One **Positive Thing** I Noticed Today . . .
2 I ate what I really wanted	
3 I ate consciously	
4 I stopped when full	
5 I drank water	What I'm **Looking Forward To** Tomorrow . . .
6 I moved my body	
7 I listened to the CD	
8 I did the mirror exercise	

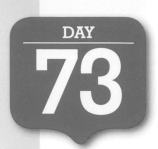
TODAY'S SUCCESS CHECKLIST

1. ☐ I ate when I was hungry

2. ☐ I ate what I really wanted

3. ☐ I ate consciously

4. ☐ I stopped when full

5. ☐ I drank water

6. ☐ I moved my body

7. ☐ I listened to the CD

8. ☐ I did the mirror exercise

One **Positive Thing**
I Noticed Today . . .

....

....

....

What I'm **Looking Forward To**
Tomorrow . . .

....

....

....

Q: After I finish the 90-day programme, can I go back to weighing myself every day?

By weighing yourself daily, you're just guaranteeing yourself frustration – up one day and down the next. In fact, your weight can fluctuate up to five pounds every single day regardless of how much or how little you eat.

In any case, I believe your weight is the least important measurement of progress you can make. Try these on for size instead:

1 How comfortable do your clothes feel on you?

2 How comfortable do you feel in yourself?

As long as you're feeling better and your clothes are feeling looser, you're making progress!

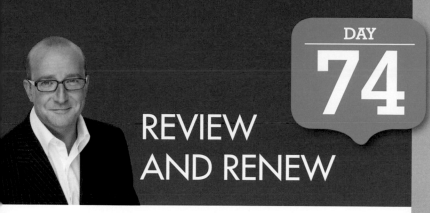

74

REVIEW AND RENEW

TODAY'S SUCCESS CHECKLIST

☐ 1 I ate when I was hungry

☐ 2 I ate what I really wanted

☐ 3 I ate consciously

☐ 4 I stopped when full

☐ 5 I drank water

☐ 6 I moved my body

☐ 7 I listened to the CD

☐ 8 I did the mirror exercise

SO LONG AS A PERSON IS CAPABLE OF SELF-RENEWAL, THEY ARE A LIVING BEING.

HENRI FRÉDÉRIC AMIEL

Hopefully, you've already realized that the best answers to your questions are the ones you give yourself.

Today, give yourself the gift of going through the review process in more detail than you normally do – you may be surprised by what you discover!

1. The best things that happened this week were:

....

2. My biggest challenges this week were:

....

3. I did these things for the first time:

....

4. What I learned was:

....

5. My top three priorities for the week ahead are:

a. ....

b. ....

c. ....

One **Positive Thing**
I Noticed Today . . .

....

....

What I'm **Looking Forward To**
Tomorrow . . .

....

....

....

233

DAY
75

YOUR FIFTH CHECK-IN . . .

THE FIRST AND WORST OF ALL FRAUDS IS TO CHEAT YOURSELF.

PEARL BAILEY

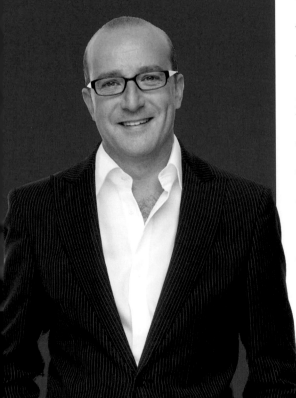

TODAY I WEIGH

As you reflect back over the past weeks and months, you can no doubt point to one or two key moments when you made a breakthrough decision or did something for the first time that let you know you really have changed.

Take some time today to acknowledge those moments, and in particular to acknowledge yourself for everything you've done to change your life for the better . . .

My 'breakthrough' moments:

1. What happened:

....

....

What changed:

....

....

2. What happened:

....

....

What changed:

....

....

3. What happened:

....

....

What changed:

....

....

KATE HOWLETT

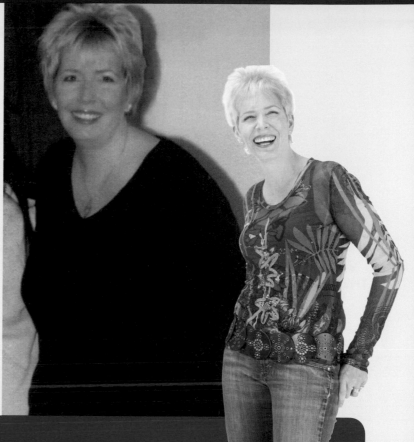

LOST 5½ STONE

KATE'S STORY

I had tried every sort of diet: fat counting, calorie counting, I even tried never eating before 5pm. I had finally given up. I was fat. It ran in my family. There was nothing I could do. Then a colleague told me she'd followed the Paul McKenna system and she was feeling great, so I gave it a try.

I was amazed. It's actually easy to lose weight. I realized that this system was not a diet but a new way of looking at food. Now I enjoy my food, instead of spending all my time thinking about it and then wolfing it down thoughtlessly. The only problem is in restaurants, where the portions are too big and I have to explain that the food was good but there was just too much of it.

I still listen to the CD. It says I'll have more energy on waking up – and I do. I walk my son to school now; I always used to take the car. I love shopping for clothes, which I used to dread. Since doing the Paul McKenna system, I feel much more positive about life. In a way, the weight loss is just a bonus!

> **VICTORY BELONGS TO THE MOST PERSEVERING.**
> — NAPOLEON

WEEK 11

INTO THE HOME STRETCH

DAY 76

FINISH WHAT YOU STARTED

What do you need to do to feel you gave your all to this programme?

As we come into the final two weeks of our time together, I hope you'll consider what it would take to make sure that whatever the outcome, you feel great about your part in making this 90-day journal a true success.

Today, renew your commitment to living each of the four golden keys to permanent weight loss:

1 When you are hungry, EAT.

2 EAT WHAT YOU WANT,
   not what you think you should.

3 Eat CONSCIOUSLY and
   enjoy every mouthful.

4 When you think you are full, STOP eating.

Make the next two weeks your best ones yet!

TODAY'S SUCCESS CHECKLIST

1 ☐ I ate when I was hungry

2 ☐ I ate what I really wanted

3 ☐ I ate consciously

4 ☐ I stopped when full

5 ☐ I drank water

6 ☐ I moved my body

7 ☐ I listened to the CD

8 ☐ I did the mirror exercise

One **Positive Thing**
I Noticed Today . . .

What I'm **Looking Forward To**
Tomorrow . . .

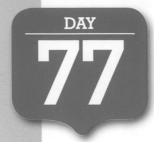
IT'S NOT THAT I'M SO SMART – IT'S JUST THAT I STAY WITH PROBLEMS LONGER.
ALBERT EINSTEIN

TODAY'S SUCCESS CHECKLIST

1 I ate when I was hungry

2 I ate what I really wanted

3 I ate consciously

4 I stopped when full

5 I drank water

6 I moved my body

7 I listened to the CD

8 I did the mirror exercise

One **Positive Thing** I Noticed Today . . .

What I'm **Looking Forward To** Tomorrow . . .

CLEARING THE WAY

In 1908, during the aftermath of the Russo-Japanese war which saw more Japanese ships sunk by floating mines than by any other offensive weapon, the British Royal Navy began developing gunboats, fishing trawlers and even private fishing boats into what became known as 'mine sweepers' – specially outfitted ships that could move slowly through enemy waters to locate and destroy mines. Once the mines were cleared, supply ships and additional troops could then be passed through the cleared area to carry out their mission at a much faster rate.

Why the impromptu history lesson?

Because many of the problems you might face over the next few months are predictable, and therefore avoidable.

Take some time today to look around your life for 'pre-problems' – those things which, if you don't take action on them soon, are liable to become a problem two or three steps further down the line. These might include an unresolved disagreement with a colleague or friend, an insurance policy whose premiums have lapsed or an unidentified ache or pain that 'isn't quite bad enough to do anything about'.

When you find a pre-problem, take action today to prevent it from becoming a 'real' problem in the future!

DAY 78

SELF-INTIMACY

MY FRIENDS TELL ME I HAVE AN INTIMACY PROBLEM. BUT THEY DON'T REALLY KNOW ME.

GARRY SHANDLING

One of the 'hidden' benefits of working through this programme is that you've probably been learning more about yourself than ever before.

And that kind of self-intimacy is a precious gift.

Today, I'd like you to up your time in the mirror – spend at least ten minutes with yourself and your body. You don't have to 'do' anything – just see what you see, feel what you feel and stay present with yourself and the process throughout.

Write down what you noticed in the space below:

....

....

....

....

....

....

....

....

TODAY'S SUCCESS CHECKLIST

1 I ate when I was hungry

2 I ate what I really wanted

3 I ate consciously

4 I stopped when full

5 I drank water

6 I moved my body

7 I listened to the CD

8 I did the mirror exercise

One **Positive Thing**
I Noticed Today . . .

What I'm **Looking Forward To**
Tomorrow . . .

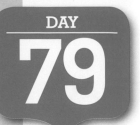
IF WE ARE FACING IN THE RIGHT DIRECTION, ALL WE HAVE TO DO IS KEEP ON WALKING.

BUDDHIST PROVERB

TODAY'S SUCCESS CHECKLIST

- [1] I ate when I was hungry
- [2] I ate what I really wanted
- [3] I ate consciously
- [4] I stopped when full
- [5] I drank water
- [6] I moved my body
- [7] I listened to the CD
- [8] I did the mirror exercise

One **Positive Thing**
I Noticed Today . . .

....

....

What I'm **Looking Forward To**
Tomorrow . . .

....

....

....

A SIMPLE RECIPE (FOR SUCCESS)

Make a list of what's been moving you towards your goals for this programme and what's been taking you away from them.

What's been moving me towards my goals:

....

....

....

....

....

What been taking me away from my goals:

....

....

....

....

....

Your assignment today is simple – do more of everything on your first list and less of everything on your second!

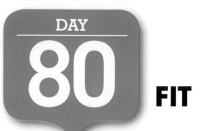

DAY 80

FIT FOR LIFE

IF IT WEREN'T FOR THE FACT THAT THE TV SET AND THE REFRIGERATOR ARE SO FAR APART, SOME OF US WOULDN'T GET ANY EXERCISE AT ALL. JOEY ADAMS

Here is an amazingly simple programme you can use as an aid to fat burning. It will take you about 10 minutes to do, can be done anywhere and needs no special equipment . . .

1 For the first minute or so, get your body moving slowly. You can use any form of gentle stretch – it should feel easy and natural, like a cat getting up from an afternoon nap.

2 For the next phase, aim to do at least five push-ups and five stomach crunches as slowly as possible. See if you can count to 10 on the way up and another 10 on the way down. If regular push-ups are too hard for you, begin the push-ups on your knees or even by pushing away against a wall until you become stronger.)

3 For the third and final part of this routine, you can use virtually any activity that causes your body to breathe more deeply and your heart rate to quicken. Walking, dancing, swimming, even climbing stairs will work perfectly well – of course, you can always use a treadmill, stair climber or exercise bike if you prefer. There are two easy rules to follow – keep moving for a full five minutes, and if the exercise feels too hard, slow down; if it feels too easy, speed up!

TODAY'S SUCCESS CHECKLIST

1 I ate when I was hungry

2 I ate what I really wanted

3 I ate consciously

4 I stopped when full

5 I drank water

6 I moved my body

7 I listened to the CD

8 I did the mirror exercise

One **Positive Thing** I Noticed Today . . .

What I'm **Looking Forward To** Tomorrow . . .

TODAY'S SUCCESS CHECKLIST

1. ☐ I ate when I was hungry

2. ☐ I ate what I really wanted

3. ☐ I ate consciously

4. ☐ I stopped when full

5. ☐ I drank water

6. ☐ I moved my body

7. ☐ I listened to the CD

8. ☐ I did the mirror exercise

One **Positive Thing**
I Noticed Today . . .

What I'm **Looking Forward To**
Tomorrow . . .

DAY 81

SUCCESS HIGHLIGHT FILMS

THE SECRET OF SUCCESS IS CONSTANCY OF PURPOSE.

BENJAMIN DISRAELI

In my book **Instant Confidence**, I share this powerful technique you can use any time you want a boost of confidence, energy and wellbeing:

1 I'd like you imagine right now that you are watching a movie about a future, more successful you. Notice every detail of how that future you looks – the expression on your face, the way you are holding your body and the light in your eyes.

2 As the movie plays out on the screen in front of you, you will see many moments of success from your past, and others that have not yet happened. Sit back and enjoy the show!

3 When you're ready, I'd like you to float out of your seat and into that successful you up on the screen. See through their eyes, hear through their ears and feel the feelings of your successful self. Make the colours brighter, the sounds louder and the feelings stronger.

4 Notice where that feeling of success is strongest in your body and give it a colour. Now move that colour up to the top of your head and down to the tip of your toes, doubling the brightness and doubling it again.

5 Float back into your present moment self, being sure to keep as much of the feeling of natural confidence and success as feels truly wonderful.

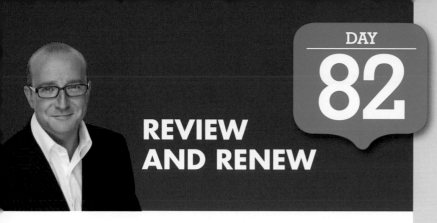

REVIEW AND RENEW

TODAY'S SUCCESS CHECKLIST

1 ☐ I ate when I was hungry

2 ☐ I ate what I really wanted

3 ☐ I ate consciously

4 ☐ I stopped when full

5 ☐ I drank water

6 ☐ I moved my body

7 ☐ I listened to the CD

8 ☐ I did the mirror exercise

IF A MAN DOES HIS BEST, WHAT ELSE IS THERE?

GENERAL GEORGE S. PATTON

As you prepare for our final week together, take the time to review, renew and celebrate how far you've come. This will allow you to enter into the final week with what Zen monks call 'beginner's mind' – the ability to live each moment as if it is your first . . .

1. The best things that happened this week were:

....

2. My biggest challenges this week were:

....

3. I did these things for the first time:

....

4. What I learned was:

....

5. My top three priorities for the week ahead are:

a.
....

b.
....

c.
....

One **Positive Thing**
I Noticed Today . . .

....

....

What I'm **Looking Forward To**
Tomorrow . . .

....

....

....

SUCCESS IS NOT A PLACE AT WHICH ONE ARRIVES, BUT RATHER THE SPIRIT WITH WHICH ONE UNDERTAKES AND CONTINUES THE JOURNEY.

ALEX NOBLE

WEEK 12

A NEW BEGINNING

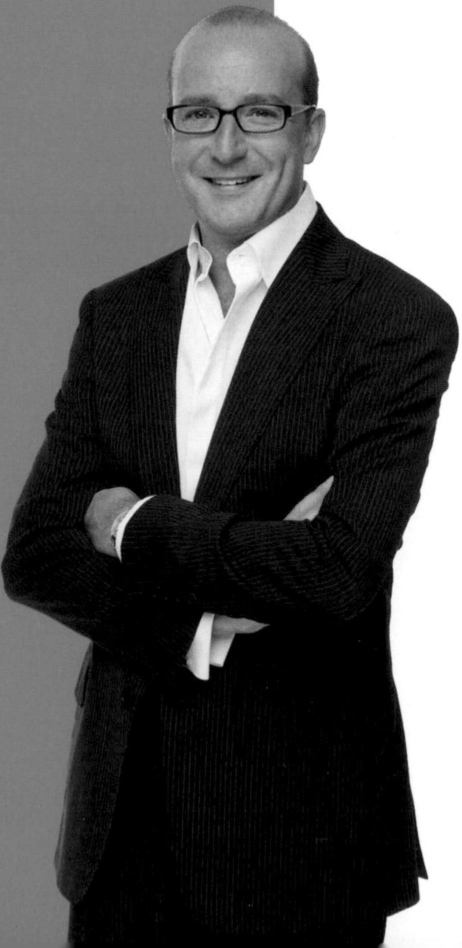

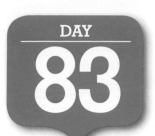

**THE MOST IMPORTANT
CHOICE YOU MAKE IS WHAT
YOU CHOOSE TO MAKE
IMPORTANT.**
MICHAEL NEILL

THERE'S MORE TO LIFE THAN BEING THIN!

What would you do if the world was going to end one week from today? In his book **The Power of Full Engagement**, corporate coach Dr James Loehr offers the following questions to help you get in touch with your core values – the most important things in your world:

1 Jump ahead to the end of your life. What are the three most important lessons you have learned and why are they so critical?

....

....

2 Think of someone you deeply respect. Describe three qualities in this person that you most admire.

....

....

3 Who are you at your best?

....

....

4 What one-sentence inscription would you like to see on your tombstone that would capture who you really were in your life?

....

....

TODAY'S SUCCESS CHECKLIST

1 I ate when I was hungry

2 I ate what I really wanted

3 I ate consciously

4 I stopped when full

5 I drank water

6 I moved my body

7 I listened to the CD

8 I did the mirror exercise

One **Positive Thing**
I Noticed Today . . .

What I'm **Looking Forward To**
Tomorrow . . .

AH BUT A MAN'S REACH
SHOULD EXCEED HIS GRASP,
ELSE WHAT'S A HEAVEN FOR?
ROBERT BROWNING

**TODAY'S SUCCESS
CHECKLIST**

1 I ate when I was hungry

2 I ate what I really wanted

3 I ate consciously

4 I stopped when full

5 I drank water

6 I moved my body

7 I listened to the CD

8 I did the mirror exercise

One **Positive Thing**
I Noticed Today . . .

What I'm **Looking Forward To**
Tomorrow . . .

A VISION FOR YOUR FUTURE

What is your vision for the future? In other words, how would you like your life to be in 5, 10, 15 or even 20 years from now? Take some time today to dream. Here are some questions from **Change Your Life in 7 Days** to get you started . . .

- **If you could be, do or have anything you want, what would you love to be, do and have?**

- **What would you choose to do if you had unlimited resources?**

- **What would you love to give back to the world?**

- **What would you attempt if you knew you could not fail?**

Jot down some ideas for your vision in the space below. Tomorrow, I'll share with you one of my favourite ways of turning your ideas into a vivid vision your unconscious will find it impossible to ignore:

DAY 85
YOUR IDEAL WEEK

YOUR VISION WILL BECOME CLEAR ONLY WHEN YOU LOOK INTO YOUR HEART. WHO LOOKS OUTSIDE, DREAMS. WHO LOOKS INSIDE, AWAKENS.

CARL JUNG

Today, I want you to review your notes from yesterday and write out what an ideal week might be like in your future . . .

- **How does your week begin?**
- **How good do you feel?**
- **Where do you go each day?**
- **What do you do?**
- **Who do you spend your time with?**
- **What lets you know how wonderful your life has become?**

On Monday, I . . .

On Tuesday, I . . .

On Wednesday, I . . . etc

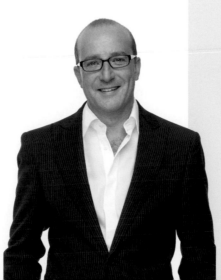

TODAY'S SUCCESS CHECKLIST

1. I ate when I was hungry

2. I ate what I really wanted

3. I ate consciously

4. I stopped when full

5. I drank water

6. I moved my body

7. I listened to the CD

8. I did the mirror exercise

One **Positive Thing** I Noticed Today . . .

What I'm **Looking Forward To** Tomorrow . . .

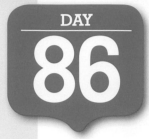
IT DOESN'T MATTER WHAT
WE DO UNTIL WE ACCEPT
OURSELVES. ONCE WE ACCEPT
OURSELVES, IT DOESN'T MATTER
WHAT WE DO.
CHARLY HEAVENRICH

FAT IS NOT A FEELING

Chances are that even after all this time, you may still have days where you hear yourself say, 'I feel fat!' What's important to know is this:

Fat is not a feeling – it's a perception.

If today is a 'fat day', don't adjust your diet – adjust your attitude. Because if you're 'feeling' fat, chances are there's something else you're not allowing yourself to feel . . .

1 Tune into your body, particularly the area between your neck and your pelvis.

2 Allow yourself just to be with whatever is going on in your body for at least 30 seconds.

3 When you're ready, let it go. Take at least 30 seconds more to imagine any uncomfortable feelings leaving your body and disappearing into the earth or sky.

4 Now think about someone or something you love and someone or something that loves you. Think about something you're grateful for in your life.

5 When you're feeling more centred and at peace, return to your day refreshed!

TODAY'S SUCCESS CHECKLIST

- [1] I ate when I was hungry
- [2] I ate what I really wanted
- [3] I ate consciously
- [4] I stopped when full
- [5] I drank water
- [6] I moved my body
- [7] I listened to the CD
- [8] I did the mirror exercise

One **Positive Thing**
I Noticed Today . . .

What I'm **Looking Forward To**
Tomorrow . . .

DAY 87

YOUR KEYS TO SUCCESS

LOVE IS THE MASTER KEY WHICH OPENS THE GATES TO HAPPINESS.

OLIVER WENDELL HOLMES

A friend of mine was telling me about the moment when he first handed his daughter the keys to the family car and waved a tearful goodbye as she drove down the road on her own for the first time. He knew that for the first time what mattered now was not how much he knew about driving, but how much she had been able to learn.

In a similar way, I have now shared with you the best of what I've learned about how anyone can feel great, lose weight and keep it off for life. Today, begin to turn my system into your system by writing down your keys to success – the things you have discovered over the past few months which really make the difference between failure and success for YOU . . .

My Keys to Success:

1.
2.
3.
4.
5.

TODAY'S SUCCESS CHECKLIST

1. ☐ I ate when I was hungry

2. ☐ I ate what I really wanted

3. ☐ I ate consciously

4. ☐ I stopped when full

5. ☐ I drank water

6. ☐ I moved my body

7. ☐ I listened to the CD

8. ☐ I did the mirror exercise

One **Positive Thing** I Noticed Today . . .

What I'm **Looking Forward To** Tomorrow . . .

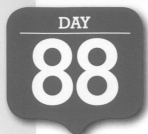

WHAT'S NEXT?

1. I ate when I was hungry

2. I ate what I really wanted

3. I ate consciously

4. I stopped when full

5. I drank water

6. I moved my body

7. I listened to the CD

8. I did the mirror exercise

One **Positive Thing**
I Noticed Today . . .

What I'm **Looking Forward To**
Tomorrow . . .

CHANGE STARTS WHEN SOMEONE SEES THE NEXT STEP.

WILLIAM DRAYTON

The question I am asked most frequently when people have successfully completed one of my programmes is, 'What's next?'

Now that you have successfully taken yourself through this programme, there is one thing you can do which more than any other will help you to build on the momentum you've generated and keep your relationship with eating, food and your body strong: volunteer your support for other people who want to lose weight!

Chances are that people have already begun asking you what you're doing differently. Instead of just telling them, you can show them. Take them through the four golden rules. Share the secrets of easy exercise. Encourage them to work through this programme with you as a 'support coach'.

Not only will they thank you, your mastery of the system will grow in leaps and bounds, and you will find it easier and easier to maintain all the gains (and losses!) you have made!

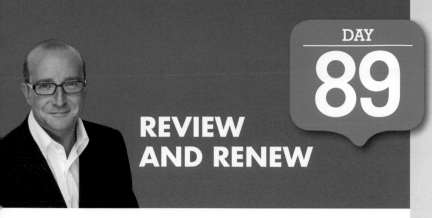

REVIEW AND RENEW

TODAY'S SUCCESS CHECKLIST

[1] I ate when I was hungry

[2] I ate what I really wanted

[3] I ate consciously

[4] I stopped when full

[5] I drank water

[6] I moved my body

[7] I listened to the CD

[8] I did the mirror exercise

IT'S LACK OF FAITH THAT MAKES PEOPLE AFRAID OF MEETING CHALLENGES, AND I BELIEVE IN MYSELF. MUHAMMAD ALI

Did you really believe when you embarked on this journal that you would make it all the way to the end? Whether or not you did, you can certainly believe in yourself now – and you will find that your belief in yourself is one of the most powerful tools for creating lasting changes in your life. The next time you find yourself face to face with a challenge, you will be able to look it straight in the eye and say to yourself in your most confident voice, 'I can do this!'

Take some time today to once again review the week gone by and to look ahead to the next:

1. The best things that happened this week were:

2. My biggest challenges this week were:

3. I did these things for the first time:

4. What I learned was:

5. My top three priorities for the week ahead are:

a.

b.

c.

One **Positive Thing** I Noticed Today . . .

What I'm **Looking Forward To** Tomorrow . . .

251

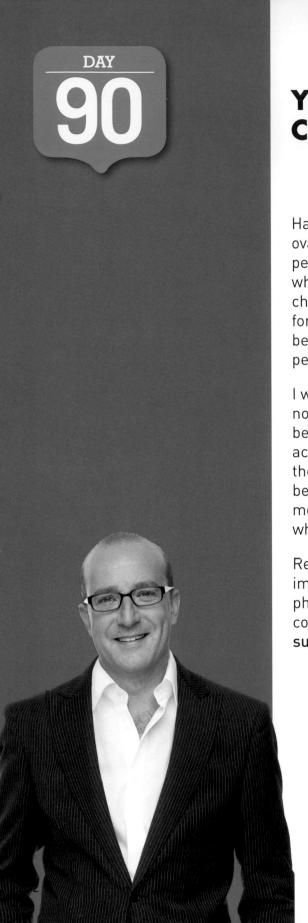

DAY
90

YOUR LAST CHECK-IN . . .

Have you ever seen a performer get a standing ovation? As the applause begins, one or two people stand, then a few more, and soon the whole audience is on its feet, stamping and cheering and applauding out of complete respect for the performer and gratitude for having been able in some small way to be a part of the performance.

I want you to know that if I was there with you now, I would be leading the applause and I would be the very first person to stand! What you have accomplished is phenomenal – and perhaps the best thing of all is that 90 days after you've begun, you don't need me to tell you that any more. You know beyond a shadow of a doubt that what you've achieved is yours to keep forever.

Remember, today's testimonial is the most important one of all – yours! Be sure to get a photo done and paste it into the slot. Send your completed testimonial with photos to **success@mckenna.com**.

SUCCESS STORIES

PLACE YOUR
BEFORE IMAGE HERE

PLACE YOUR
AFTER IMAGE HERE

YOUR NAME:

....

....

YOUR STORY

I LOST

STONE

....

....

....

....

....

....

....

....

....

INDEX OF TECHNIQUES

ACKNOWLEDGEMENTS

I would like to thank Dr Hugh Willbourn, Dr Ronald Ruden, Dr Richard Bandler, Dr Roger Callahan, Dr Natheera Indrasanen, and all the people who have used and supported this system over the years by sharing their success stories in writing or even by walking up to me on the street. You have inspired so many others over the planet through your generosity of spirit.

More than any of my other books, this beautiful colour extended version is the collective vision of a group of very talented people: Alex Tuppen, Doug Young, Mari Roberts and Michael Neill. It's a privilege working with you!

WOULD YOU LIKE TO WORK WITH PAUL MCKENNA AS YOUR PERSONAL WEIGHT LOSS COACH?

HOW MUCH MORE SUCCESSFUL DO YOU THINK YOU COULD BE IN REACHING YOUR GOALS?

As an additional resource for readers of this book, Paul has now created a membership website at **www.mckenna.com** where you can get complete support in reaching your weight-loss goals.

Here is just some of what you get:

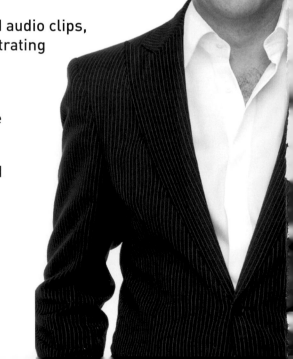

- A 14-day jumpstart programme customized to your personal weight-loss needs

- Members-only access to Paul's regular podcast where you can call and talk with him directly about your personal weight-loss issues

- Access to an online library of video and audio clips, including mini-movies of Paul demonstrating every technique in this book

- Daily tips and exclusive advice from bestselling author and life coach to the Hollywood elite, Michael Neill

- A sense of belonging, camaraderie and friendship with other members of one of the largest online weight-loss communities in the world!

To join the club and learn more, visit **www.mckenna.com**